MINDING YOUR BODY

ALSO BY JOSEPH S. RECHTSCHAFFEN, M.D., AND ROBERT CAROLA

Dr. Rechtschaffen's Diet for
Lifetime Weight Control and Better Health
(updated edition)

MINDING YOUR BODY

100 Ways to Live and Be Well

JOSEPH S. RECHTSCHAFFEN, M.D.,
AND ROBERT CAROLA

With original recipes by Ann Seranne

Foreword by Donna Karan

KODANSHA INTERNATIONAL
New York • Tokyo • London

Kodansha America, Inc.
114 Fifth Avenue, New York, New York 10011, U.S.A.

Kodansha International Ltd.
17-14 Otowa 1-chome, Bunkyo-ku, Tokyo 112, Japan

Published in 1995 by Kodansha America, Inc.

LIBRARY OF CONGRESS CATALOGING-IN-PUBLICATION DATA
Rechtschaffen, Joseph S.
    Minding your body : 100 ways to live and be well /
Joseph S. Rechtschaffen and Robert Carola.
        p.   cm.
    Includes index.
    ISBN 1-56836-076-2
    1. Nutrition. 2. Health. 3. Exercise. 4. Weight loss. I. Carola,
Robert. II. Title.
RA784.R432   1995   95-3823
613—dc20

Book design by Laura Lindgren

Printed in the United States of America

95 96 97 98 99   Q/FF   10 9 8 7 6 5 4 3 2 1

This book is dedicated to our wives,
Fran Rechtschaffen and Leslie Conron Carola

◆ ◆

We should set the highest value, not on living, but on living well.
—SOCRATES, "CRITO"

Most folks are about as happy as they make up their minds to be.
—ABRAHAM LINCOLN

God gave us burdens, also shoulders.
—YIDDISH PROVERB

◆ ◆

CONTENTS

---

100 WAYS TO LIVE AND BE WELL

To live and be well . . .

◆ ◆ ◆

FOREWORD

Anne Klein not only gave me my start in fashion, she gave me my start in healthy living as well. She introduced me to my doctor, Dr. Rechtschaffen, and for that I am eternally grateful. Throughout my adult life, he has been my safety net, my closest advisor, the physician I rely on. I trust him with my life.

Dr. Rechtschaffen is the kind of doctor who's not supposed to exist anymore. An old-fashioned family M.D., he's sensitive, warm, and caring. He's a rock of Gibraltar, and you can tell him absolutely anything. He's also my husband's primary physician, and should anyone in our company get sick, Dr. Rechtschaffen is there, willing and able. He's even been known to make house calls!

Why am I so crazy about Joe Rechtschaffen? He appreciates stress, temptation, and the many complexities of modern life. He treats the whole person, since he believes the route to a healthy body begins with a sound mind and a peaceful soul.

Dr. Rechtschaffen gave me a philosophy to live by: eat a mostly vegetarian diet with little or no salt, stay active ("Walk, walk, walk!," as he likes to say), and most important of all, trust that I'll be able to do it. There are no lectures or wagging finger when I slip up (and believe me, I do). Just understanding encouragement from a supportive confidant.

Unfortunately, all the people in the world don't live in New York City. If they did, there's a doctor I could recommend. But this book is the next best thing. Dr. Rechtschaffen has compressed the equivalent of one hundred private office visits into the pages you're holding in your hand. Read it. Cherish it. Live by it.

Donna Karan
New York City
December 1994

A WORD TO THE READER

Science and medicine have made tremendous advances. In the last seventy-five years our average life expectancy has increased from 54 to 76 years. The task for each of us is to make those extra years the healthiest, fittest they can be. The overall concern of this book is not to help you diet and lose weight, but rather to help you achieve and maintain good health to enhance the *quality of your life*. There are four ways to accomplish this:

1. Mind your body, and trust what it tells you.
2. Eat positively.
3. Be physically active.
4. Try to combat unhealthy stress by relaxing.

The first step to minding your body is knowing what your body needs in order to do the job it was meant to do. We should at least think about our bodies as much as we think about our cars. You wouldn't put junk in your gas tank, so why put it in your body? Demand the best for yourself. You are worth it.

I wrote this book, not to tell you things you already know, or to force you to do things you don't want to do, but to remind you that your body is a finely tuned instrument that *knows what it needs*. Our bodies are constantly giving us clues about what works best for us, but sometimes the clues are too subtle, and we may not hear them. Or maybe we don't really want to listen.

If I had to choose one word that epitomizes what we have to do to be healthy, it would be *activity*. And that doesn't have to be just *physical* activity. The constructive activity of our *minds* is just as important. If our minds are active, looking for things to explore, our bodies will be active, too. Being active is the only way to keep our bodies healthy. We were not meant to sit still and daydream. We were meant to use our bodies *and* our minds.

With regular, consistent physical and mental activity you will find that your body will naturally seek a healthy balance. The cravings you had for fat-laden foods will lessen, overeating of fatty foods will be a thing of the past, your mind will be clearer, you will be more productive, your mood will improve, and sleep will be more restful.

Late in 1994 researchers at the Rockefeller University in New York City discovered a mutated gene that may be responsible for causing obesity in some people. The faulty gene, labeled the "obesity gene," is believed to disrupt both the body's metabolism and its appetite control center, making it difficult for a person with the gene to recognize the typical signs of fullness or satisfaction. So a person with a faulty obesity gene goes right on eating after the body has accumulated enough food. But the researchers warn that their study, which was conducted on mice, is a long way from being applicable to people and solving the problem of human obesity. In the meantime, I continue to recommend a healthy diet and lots of physical activity.

I have been a physician for more than forty-five years, and nothing has been more satisfying than witnessing individuals commit themselves to maintaining a healthy lifestyle. Give your body a chance to find its own proper level, its own balance, and it will. It makes much more sense to try to prevent disease than to try to cure it.

Read this book with the understanding that what I offer you here is what I would say to you if you were in my office. The principles in this book are those that I've been telling my patients for years and have been practicing myself for a lifetime.

IMPROVE THE QUALITY OF YOUR LIFE

The truth is, all of life's difficulties are easier to handle when we feel healthy and are healthy because we are in good physical and mental condition. We can feel that our bodies and our minds are together, on the same wavelength. It's always easier to face life when you meet it with the physical and emotional energy that flows from a feeling of wellbeing.

We have to go on living, easy or not, and we might as well make the most of life. One of the most important qualities to nurture in ourselves is the ability to *change*, to adapt to the world around us and within us. Why not enjoy life?

With this book, I hope to convince you to improve the quality of your life by becoming mentally and physically fit. Money doesn't necessarily improve the quality of our lives, but good health does.

IS THERE A QUICK FIX?

Am I going to propose ideas that are quick and easy? Absolutely not. But compared with other approaches that only lead to frustration—with endless cycles of stress, illness, weight gain, dieting, and all the rest—the positive ideas in this book *are* relatively simple, because they are connected to your body's own balanced needs. As you'll find, your body responds quickly to positive ideas.

This book is going to help you listen to your body and respond positively to what you hear.

YOUR BODY ALREADY KNOWS
MOST OF THE ANSWERS

Your body is a sophisticated entity that knows what it needs. It has been designed to be in a *state of balance*—never too much or too little of anything. Haven't you ever felt that your body was trying to tell you what to eat or what type of physical activity to do? This happens all the time, but we often ignore the signals. Listen to your body, and mind what it tells you.

AVOID FRUSTRATION, BUT DON'T
UNDERESTIMATE YOURSELF

I wrote this book to help you, not to complicate your life or add to the many everyday pressures you already feel. If we are to improve the quality of our lives, we must feel good about ourselves. There's no point in asking for the impossible, but there's also no point in underestimating what *is* possible. Above all, don't put yourself in a position where the only possible outcome is frustration. You can do what is best for you. You won't *want* to do anything less.

THIS BOOK IS EASY TO READ,
THE RECIPES ARE EASY TO USE

This book has been designed for easy reading, one point at a time. Instead of lengthy chapters, there are one or two pages for each of the "100 Ways to Live and Be Well." In the process, I talk about the things that are important to you, sometimes with new information and sometimes with reminders of what you already know but may have forgotten—things that bear repeating within this context so you can see the whole picture. We should always keep the whole picture in mind.

The short, nontechnical appendices offer useful information about food, food labels, vitamins, and minerals. The book concludes with some of my favorite recipes—ones that anybody can handle. I'm not expecting you to be a gourmet chef, or even to have the *time* to be a gourmet chef. The recipes are basic ones that you can personalize and vary easily. They were chosen to make mealtimes easier for you, and they will help you start applying the idea of *positive eating*.

When you apply the principles in this book, know that you're doing something that is good for *you*. You're concentrating on *doing what is good for you,* instead of on not doing what is bad for you. Once you understand and believe this point, you really won't have to think about it all the time. It becomes part of a common-sense attitude that is a *natural, balanced* way of living. (Now read that paragraph again—it's important.)

HOW THE ESSAYS ARE ORGANIZED

The publisher and I gave a great deal of thought to the format of the book, and as stated earlier, I finally decided on short, easy-to-absorb essays. One thing at a time, and one step at a time, is more important and sensible than trying to do everything at once.

I hope you will read each section as a separate tip on how to live and be well—as if each essay was the theme of an office consultation between you and me. In fact, it might be a good idea to think of my book as a series of "office visits," to be read and thought about one at a time, instead of reading the whole book from cover to cover in one sitting.

Rather than placing all the essays on one subject (physical activity, for example) together, I have distributed them throughout the book so you do not have to read all about one subject at the same time. I hope this arrangement will make your reading more pleasant. Also, I have repeated some points occasionally, when I thought they were important enough to reinforce. Check the table of contents and the index for specific topics you may be interested in.

WE ARE IN THIS TOGETHER

Remember that I would never ask you to do something that I would not do (or have not done) myself. I try to practice what I preach, and you should too. Setting a good example is the best way to teach a way of life.

So please, when you read this book, try to think of it as a conversation between you and me. I will be there to support you every step of the way.

AT LEAST WE CAN MAKE LIFE EASIER

I hope my suggestions, based on my forty-five years' experience as a physician, will help you find something that will change your life for the better. Life is not always easy, but you can make it *easier*. Give it a chance.

Joseph S. Rechtschaffen, M.D.

New York City

December 1994

ACKNOWLEDGMENTS

The authors would like to express their gratitude to the following people: Peggy Gallagher, Barbara Blakemore, Carolyn Blakemore, Craig Claiborne, Adi Giovannetti, Irwin Glusker, Donna Karan, Stephan Rechtschaffen, M.D., Michael Tong, our literary agents F. Joseph Spieler and Lisa M. Ross, and the staff of Kodansha America, especially Paul De Angelis, Gillian Jolis, Akiko Takano, and Maya Rao.

The suggestions in this book are not meant to replace the personalized advice of your physician. It is important to check with your physician before undertaking any dietary or physical activity program.

100 WAYS TO LIVE AND BE WELL

Listen to Your Body

Your body is designed to keep a steady, healthy balance. Every organ, every cell has ways of keeping your body from straying too far off course. Think about your body temperature. How many days of the year does it go more than 1 or 2 degrees above or below 98.6 F? And yet the temperature outside may vary 70 degrees or more during the year.

Everything about your body is aimed at constancy. Once your body has reached a level of good health, it wants to remain there. Your body can put up with external changes, like changes in the weather, but it cannot tolerate unhealthy internal changes. The condition of healthy constancy is called *homeostasis* (ho-mee-oh-STAY-siss, which comes from a Greek word that means "staying the same").

Hans Selye, a pioneer in stress research, has said in his book *The Stress of Life* that "the great capacity for *adaptation* is what makes life possible on all levels of complexity. It is the basis for homeostasis and of resistance to stress. . . . Adaptability is probably the most distinctive characteristic of life."

Your body is geared to fight changes that make it unhealthy. If you cut your finger, your body has ways to stop the bleeding and heal the wound. If you eat too many sour apples, your body will secrete the necessary chemicals to ease your stomachache.

Your body seeks a *balance* in everything you do—that's what homeostasis is all about. You can gain that balance by practicing moderation and by learning the nuances of how your body responds to certain situations, foods, and places. Learn not to push your body to its limits all the time.

One of the great, apparently hidden secrets of good health is this: *Listen to your body, and respect what it tells you.* Your body is an expert in self-preservation. It demands to be kept healthy through a balanced, moderate way of living.

One of my patients gets a headache when she takes aspirin. I don't tell her she's a hypochondriac, because she isn't. I tell her to listen to her body and take a different painkiller or maybe even to take a walk instead of a pill. Another patient says he has found a magical weight-loss food—a black-peppercorn dressing that he uses as a dip with raw cauliflower. Even though the dressing contains sour cream and mayonnaise, he swears he loses weight every time he eats it. I tell him to go ahead and eat it if it makes him lose weight and feel better. (Could it be the spicy pepper and Worcestershire sauce in the dip that promote weight loss? Or could it be that the spiciness goes a long way, and he is eating very little of it—less than he realizes—but plenty of the fiber-rich cauliflower?) When something works for you without harming you, I say, Why not?

The great sixteenth-century French essayist Montaigne said, "Let us give Nature a chance; she knows her business better than we do."

Use the Power
of Positive Eating

People who go on "weight-loss diets" may lose weight initially, but they don't keep it off. Such people usually lose the pleasure of eating because they avoid so many types of food. Eventually, feeling deprived, they return to that source of pleasure they know so well: overeating. Not just eating, mind you, but *overeating*. When something is taken away from you, you want it more than ever. And once you have it back, you overdo it.

You can keep the pleasure of eating good food and still keep fit and trim. How? Through *positive eating*—concentrating on the foods you *should* eat instead of constantly reminding yourself of what you shouldn't eat. Actually, there is no food you shouldn't eat. There is no food you have to give up entirely. You can fit any food into a healthy eating plan, at least occasionally, if you remember that moderation is the key.

If you begin a meal by looking down at your plate and hating what you see, you won't enjoy the meal or get its full nutritional benefits. So you lose both ways. How could you possibly live that way?

If you live by strict "dieting," you are bound to feel guilty when you have that occasional Tootsie Roll. So in this scenario you feel either guilty or deprived. A "diet" won't make you happy, because it emphasizes foods that you had to give up. But good-tasting, good-looking, healthy food makes you feel good because you enjoy it *without feeling guilty or deprived.* And that's the essence of positive eating: Eat three full meals a day, and *enjoy what you eat.* Be happy and free from guilt. Just don't eat junk that's going to make you unhealthy.

There is a catch to all this talk about enjoying your food, but it's a catch you can sidestep easily. Food manufacturers and advertisers know that you want to get pleasure from eating, so they are determined to seduce you with ad campaigns that say, "Eat it. It's fun. You *deserve* it." The emphasis has been shifted from "Watch your weight" to "Eating is supposed to be fun, so go ahead and enjoy yourself. And by the way, our product is *good* for you." But as with many seductions, the promise is sometimes more than the reality. Food company executives would like you to stop looking at labels so closely. Then you wouldn't see that the taste has been "improved" by adding salt, sugar, or fat. There are plenty of good foods that don't need any "taste enhancers."

Here's a hard fact from real life: In 1993 Häagen-Dazs ice cream introduced five new flavors, all with more fat and calories than their usual ice cream (which was already high in fat and calories). What happened to sales? They increased. So did your waistlines and cholesterol levels.

For a long time now you've been thinking about what *not* to eat. Now you can start thinking about what *to* eat. Think of the word *diet* in its larger sense—as an eating plan, not as a weight-loss plan. The best eating plan is a healthy one that includes foods from the three main food groups in the proper proportion. Of your total daily food intake (by weight), no more than 20 percent should be fat; 50 to 70 percent, complex carbohydrates; and 15 to 20 percent, protein. Variety and quantity in our diets are critical because no one food can supply all the nutrients necessary for good health.

Later in the book I tell you not to count calories. Even though I just gave you some recommended percentages of fat, complex carbohydrates, and protein, I don't really want you to count them either. The numbers you will see throughout the book (I tried to use them sparingly) are merely guidelines you can use to check yourself. If you are eating moderate portions of the correct foods, as I outline for you, there is no need to count every gram of food you eat. If you follow my basic principles, you will see soon enough that your new lifestyle puts you right on track with the recommended dietary guidelines.

Remember, I am not strictly prescribing a weight-loss diet. (See my other book, newly revised in paperback, *Dr. Rechtschaffen's Diet for Lifetime Weight Control and Better Health,* for a weight-loss and maintenance program.) The diet I am advocating here is one you can live with throughout your life, starting today.

If you can make up your mind that being thin and healthy and *having* food is better than being fat and *craving* food, then you will make a positive move to change your lifestyle and lose weight and be healthy permanently. The idea is simple: **Your body *wants* the foods that will encourage good health, and *you* are in control of your body.**

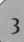

3

Stay Active Physically
and Mentally

Physical activity is not just a way to burn off calories. Regular physical activity permanently increases your metabolic rate—the rate at which your body uses energy—and allows you to burn off calories faster. A person with a high metabolic rate is burning off calories even when sitting still or sleeping. Don't you know people who seem to eat as much as they want without gaining an ounce? Those people may be eating a high-complex-carbohydrate, high-fiber diet, and what's more, they probably have a higher metabolic rate than you do. Were they born with it? Not necessarily. Remember: Your metabolic rate *can* be changed.

Traditional thinking would have you believe that you have to consciously "work off" every calorie you consume. That's just not true. Yes, you do have to use up the stored energy contained in food, but you don't have to keep a balance sheet. If your metabolic rate is high enough, your body will do the work for you. (Your metabolic rate will be high enough if you exercise regularly at least three or four times a week.) Physical activity helps regulate your appetite. If you exercise regularly, you don't really have to think about your diet.

As a rule, don't worry about calories. (You will probably end up consuming between 1,200 and 1,900 a day.) Just make a real effort to eat low-fat, high-complex-carbohydrate nutritious meals and to keep active physically. Chronic dieters live and die with calorie counting, and they ultimately discover two things: First, they get discouraged and guilt-ridden because they can't seem to be satisfied with the "proper" number of calories, which is usually far too low to be healthy anyway. Second, they gain weight no matter how hard they count calories.

Physical activity will help you feel and look better. And it will definitely help raise your metabolic rate so that *keeping* trim once you've lost weight is possible. Toned muscles burn calories faster than untoned muscles do, so strength training is another way to increase your metabolic level.

Remember that it's unnatural for us to do nothing and want nothing. We are designed for action, and our bodies and minds react positively to activity.

4

Focus on the Quality of Life

Most of us would like to be healthy and productive right up to the end of our lives. No one wants to be incapacitated, be in a hospital or nursing home, or be unable to participate in everyday living. What we do now in terms of diet, exercise, and stress reduction will affect the quality of our lives not only immediately but also twenty or thirty years down the road.

If you are in your twenties or thirties now, you may have a hard time picturing yourself in your sixties or seventies. But believe me, when you *are* sixty or seventy, you will wish you had cared for yourself a little better when you were younger. You probably have a retirement plan to take care of your "old age." So why not have a good-health plan too? *Enjoy* those final years!

We know enough about nutrition and exercise to *prevent* illness—to allow ourselves to achieve a high quality of life even in our final years. So take the time now to eat healthily, stay active, and relax.

Follow the
Eating-Right Pyramid

Here's what I have said for many years, and here's what the federal government's dietary guidelines say also:

1. Eat a variety of foods.
2. Choose a diet low in fat, saturated fat, and cholesterol.
3. Choose a diet with plenty of whole-grain products, vegetables, and fruits.
4. Use sugar, salt, and sodium-based products in moderation,
   if at all.
5. If you drink alcoholic beverages, do so in moderation.

Nutritionists from the U.S. Department of Agriculture (USDA)
have created a guide to daily food choices and planning based on
scientific data in the form of the Eating-Right Pyramid. The
pyramid divides foods into six groups, with those to be eaten most
often listed first:

Eat more
1. Bread, cereal, rice, and pasta
2. Vegetables
3. Fruits

Eat less
4. Milk, yogurt, and cheese
5. Meat, poultry, fish, dried beans, eggs, and nuts
6. Fats, oils, and sweets

These guidelines are the strongest message yet from the government to eat less fat. The pyramid indicates what research has shown to be a healthy diet built on a foundation of grains, vegetables, and fruits. Such a diet includes moderate amounts of lean meat and dairy products, and very few fats and sweets.

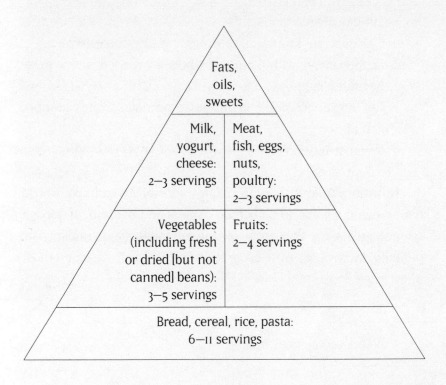

6

Seek Moderation and Balance

One of the most important concepts in being healthy is *moderation*. You have to find the balance of food intake and physical activity that you can live with. Modify any of your favorite dishes to accommodate the principles of a healthy eating and exercise plan. The way to fitness is through a healthy diet plan and a healthy physical activity program. We can all make time for these. None of us *has* the time; *make* time for it. And that's what you will do if you are serious about being the best you can be. It does feel good.

You must be prepared to make changes in your food intake and level of physical activity. But the changes will be changes that *you* choose. And this is not to say that you will never enjoy chocolate mousse cake again. You can keep eating all kinds of foods if you keep the key concepts of moderation and balance in mind. Making healthy choices helps you enjoy life.

7 ◆ Eat Less, Gain More

To eat properly, you need to avoid getting too hungry. How do you do that? By eating three meals a day. That may seem simplistic or even contradictory if you are trying to lose weight. If you skip meals with the thought that you are doing yourself a favor by eating less, you are actually doing yourself a serious injustice.

If you skip a meal, you'll be twice as hungry as you should be at your next meal, and you'll probably eat more than you should. Skipped meals can also lead to snacking, because you get too hungry to wait for mealtime. Finally, as you'll see later, when you eat less, your body metabolism slows down, making it even more difficult to keep your weight down. I *want* you to eat. Do not starve yourself, no matter what your present weight is.

Forget about being on a "diet." *Weight-loss diets don't work,* and health spas take your money and give you only short-term solutions. Save your time and money. Invest in yourself and in a healthy lifestyle you can live with—one that will keep you trim *and* healthy for as long as you live.

Recognize How Diet and Physical Activity Go Together

At least 65 percent of the people in the United States are over-weight. (By the way, I don't consider *obese* and *overweight* to mean the same thing. If you weigh more than the insurance company guidelines say, you are *overweight,* but you are not *obese* until you weigh at least 20 percent over the desirable weight.) But now, more than ever, many Americans have decided to be healthy by eating sensibly and being physically active. Everywhere you look, you see people jogging, walking, riding bikes, and skating. And many food labels read "Less fat, less sugar, less salt, more fiber!"

Yet only about one-third of American adults take part in a physical activity at least three times a week, and too many people who mean well end up only eating sensibly or only being physically active. It's easy to say, "I'm eating so sensibly that I don't need to worry about being active," or, "I'm so active I don't need to worry about what I eat." If you are overweight and you want to lose weight, such a philosophy won't work. Eventually the extra food or the lack of activity will catch up with you, and you will gain weight and feel less healthy. However, one study after another has proved that when you are physically active, you are less likely to want rich, unhealthy food.

Here are the likely outcomes if you try to lose weight by (1) just eating sensibly, (2) just exercising, or (3) eating sensibly and exercising together:

1. *Eating sensibly:* You will lose some weight but gain back much of it, or you will actually gain weight.

2. *Exercising only:* You will lose a minimal amount of weight, and you probably will keep it off as long as you continue a regular program of physical activity.

3. *Eating sensibly and exercising, too:* You will lose more weight than by only eating sensibly or only exercising, and you will keep extra weight off. Also, you will:

- look and feel healthy
- reduce the risk of breast, prostate, and colon cancer
- reduce the risk of heart attack, stroke, and diabetes
- decrease your appetite
- raise your metabolic rate
- reduce stress
- improve your sleep
- increase the efficiency of your heart and lungs
- improve your muscle strength and joint flexibility
- have a longer life with a higher quality
- increase your energy
- reduce your cholesterol levels
- increase your self-esteem
- reshape your body

That final point deserves a little more explanation. Often, a person is not more than ten pounds overweight but has a body shape that reveals body fat in all the wrong places. A combined program of positive eating and regular physical activity will help you lose body fat while toning your muscles and making you look better. Because muscle is heavier than fat you may not actually lose those ten pounds, but you will look better and be healthier.

We don't always have to lose those final ten pounds to be in better shape, inside *and* outside. Throw away your bathroom scale and concentrate on your mirror.

Here's an example: If a woman diets only to reduce a dress size, she will need to lose ten pounds. If she engages in some physical activity on a regular basis—four times a week for forty-five minutes to an hour—she will need to lose only six pounds. By combining physical activity with a low-fat diet, you will lose weight and inches, and you will definitely look trimmer.

New findings show that regular physical activity increases blood flow through your blood vessels, possibly increasing the number of your immune cells and helping to prevent cancer.

9

Change Your Metabolism

Some studies have shown that most people are actually eating less than they once did. Yet these people are continuing to gain weight. Why? Eating less than your body is used to can actually cause you to *gain* weight. I know many people who refuse to believe this simple fact. They go right on "dieting"—and gaining weight—because although they eat less, they still continue their sedentary, slow-moving ways.

The term *metabolism* is the overall term used to describe all the chemical activity taking place in our bodies. As noted earlier, our *metabolic rate* is the rate at which our bodies use energy, and not everyone has the same metabolic rate. People who have a high metabolic rate burn calories faster than people with a lower metabolic rate. Although you may think you are overweight because you were born with a low metabolic rate that causes you to burn off calories slowly, this is probably not the case. Your metabolic rate *can* be changed. *You* can change it. How? By eating, moving, and thinking positively.

When you cut down on the usual amount of food you eat, your body reacts: "Uh-oh," it observes. "Something different is going on. I'm not getting as much food as I used to. I'd better slow down the machinery to conserve energy in case there's a food shortage." In fact, your body is so well conditioned to preserve itself in times of real famine that it lowers its metabolic rate well below what is necessary to cope with a temporary food shortage. Your body doesn't know how long the food shortage will last, so it prepares for the worst, slowing itself down enough to be able to survive an extended famine.

And what happens when your body slows down? You *gain weight* because you are not only conserving your body fat to be used as an energy source but also burning off calories more slowly than you used to. That makes for a double whammy and messes up a lot of people before they know what hit them.

If you need to speed up your metabolic rate in order to lose fat and maintain a healthy weight, how do you do it? There are two healthy ways to raise your metabolic rate:

1. Eat sensibly. In other words, eat three healthy meals a day.
2. Be physically *and* mentally active. Find ways to move around, and keep your mind occupied with things that make you feel enthusiastic. Don't allow yourself to get bored.

The cells in your muscles use up more energy than the cells in your body fat, so another way to raise your metabolic level is to increase the amount of your muscle tissue and decrease your fat tissue by doing weight training (for example, with Nautilus equipment or free weights). Again, you can accomplish that goal by eating sensibly and being physically active.

People who are occupied mentally and physically are rarely bored. Develop new interests and involve yourself in them as much as you can. Spend less time thinking about your "diet," and more time being involved in something bigger than yourself. You will be more interesting, healthier, and happier. In fact, when you are mentally involved in, and excited by, your work or hobby, it will energize you.

10

Lose Weight the Best Way

If you are going to lose weight, I want you to do it just once, and in a healthy manner. There is no evidence that any weight-loss diet will help you keep weight off permanently. You cannot and should not remain on such a diet for a long time. Once you stop that kind of program, your body goes right into high gear to gain back the weight that was lost so unnaturally.

If you are determined to reach a lower, healthier weight—your *normal* weight—it is never too late to start. But you must remember that you should use healthy methods to reach a healthier weight. Here are some points to review before you try to lose weight permanently:

1. *Have a realistic goal.* Don't waste your time trying to look like a fashion model. Study your body type. Start with a goal to lose 10 percent of your weight, and then maintain that level for several months before beginning on another 10 percent (if necessary). You have a far greater chance of reaching your goal if you lose weight slowly and carefully.

2. *Change your diet slowly.* If you drastically cut your food intake, your body could react by conserving energy and burning calories more slowly. You might feel deprived, and that could lead to binge eating. Weight maintenance is more easily managed when

your body has time to adjust to each lighter stage before moving on to the next one.

3. *Start by reducing the fat in your diet.* Although some fat is needed in our diets, fat is the nutrient we need the least of. Ironically, it is usually the one we consume to excess. While you are cutting down on the fat in your diet, also try to reduce your daily caloric intake *slowly.* Retrain your taste buds to enjoy leaner, healthier foods; you'll be surprised how well your taste buds respond. The more gradual the change in your diet, the more it will feel like your natural lifestyle, and not an on-again, off-again "diet."

4. *Increase your physical activity moderately.* Regular physical activity is crucial to a weight-loss program. Physical activity by itself can promote weight loss, but when combined with a low-fat, high-complex-carbohydrate diet, the results are positive, exciting, and quickly visible. Physical activity lowers the risk of heart disease, diabetes, and high blood pressure. It improves your self-esteem and makes it easier to stick with a sensible eating and activity plan. And regular and continued physical activity keeps the weight off.

It is important to increase the level of your physical activity gradually, to prevent muscle soreness and reduce the risk of injury. The best way to lose body fat through physical activity is to exercise at a moderate intensity for as long as you feel comfortable—the longer the better. It takes twenty minutes or more to start burning body fat.

5. *Keep a diary or log of your food intake and physical activity.* Record what and how much you eat and exercise, and what the circumstances are. Also, record what makes you want to overeat or want to eat inappropriate foods, or to avoid physical activity.

Find ways to motivate yourself to cope with temptations. Keeping a log is a short-term measure (about six months) to keep you motivated and aware. After you recognize your typical pattern and are able to change it to one of positive living, you will not need the log anymore.

6. *Avoid keeping high-fat foods available.* Soon you will not *want* to keep unhealthy foods.

7. *Learn to relax.* Relaxation helps combat undue stress in your life. Learn to say no to people who demand too much of your time and energy.

8. *Join a support group* if the thought of losing weight on your own is frightening or lonely. Sometimes working with a group can bolster your efforts and meet important social needs.

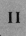

Burn Off Fat
with Aerobic Activities

Physical activity that lasts less than twenty minutes uses mostly glycogen as fuel. (Glycogen is the form of glucose stored in the muscles and liver until it is needed as a source of energy.) But any activity that takes longer than twenty minutes burns off *fat*, which is the real culprit in our diets and on our bodies. The key to fitness and good health is to drastically cut down on your intake of dietary fat and increase your participation in fat-burning activities.

Any physical activity that uses the large muscles, elevates the heart rate, and increases the need for oxygen is called *aerobic*. When you are performing an aerobic activity, you breathe hard, and you burn off fat. Through regular aerobic exercise you can safely and permanently reduce your body fat and total body weight. The longer you exercise, the more calories you burn, and the more weight and fat you lose.

When you cut down on calories, your body automatically adjusts to the lower intake, and you burn fewer calories—your metabolism slows down. But you can boost your metabolism through physical activity. Regular aerobic workouts raise your metabolic rate, so you continue to burn calories at a higher rate for several hours after you exercise.

To lose fat, the *duration* of the exercise is more important than the intensity. The best way you can lose body fat is through physical activity, which uses fat as its main source of energy. You will notice the sleeker contours of your body fairly quickly (within three to four weeks) when you participate in a regular physical activity without increasing your dietary fat intake.

Many people tend to emphasize aerobic activity to the neglect of light muscle-building activities. Aerobic activities are excellent—they will help you lose weight and be healthy—but they won't tone your muscles as well as some other activities such as rowing or using weight machines in a moderate way. Actually, *any* amount of physical activity is better than none at all. Physical activity that takes less than twenty minutes may not burn off fat, but it promotes muscle tone and will help put you in a positive frame of mind.

When we choose the right fitness program, we are helping our bodies shed the imbalance of obesity and seek a properly balanced system.

Cut through the Nutrition Confusion

Good health comes largely from eating a well-balanced diet, including foods from the three major food groups: fats, proteins, and carbohydrates. Carbohydrates supply long-term energy; proteins are the muscle-builders; and small amounts of fats are necessary to maintain healthy skin, hair, digestion, and other cellular functions. Here are some guidelines for keeping your diet well balanced.

FAT. Fat should account for no more than 20 percent of the calories you consume each day. Remember that much of the fat you eat is hidden in your food: whole milk has more fat than skim milk or low-fat milk; red meat has more fat than chicken, turkey, or fish. How you cook or prepare your food matters: frying uses more fat than grilling, broiling, steaming, or poaching; and deep-frying adds fat and calories.

PROTEIN. Protein should account for 15 to 20 percent of the calories you consume each day. Protein is found in meat, beans, wheat germ, and dairy products. If you use dairy products, concentrate on the low-fat versions.

CARBOHYDRATES. Complex carbohydrates should account for 50 to 70 percent of the calories you consume each day. Whole grains, fresh fruits, and vegetables will give you energy. They'll also help control any cravings you may have for unhealthy foods with little or no nutritional value, like candy.

SUGAR. There is no recommended level of sugar; consume limited amounts or try to avoid it altogether. Avoid sugar substitutes, which may be *carcinogenic,* or cancer causing. Remember that sweeteners such as honey and maple syrup are sugars, just like any other sugars, with no special nutritional or "natural" food value.

SODIUM. Keep your intake of sodium below 2,000 milligrams a day. Avoid salt substitutes; use herbs and spices instead. Remember that "sea salt" is no different from any other salt.

FIBER. You should consume at least 20 to 35 grams of fiber a day. Fresh vegetables and fruits are an excellent source of fiber.

Accept Problem Solving as Natural

When natural, everyday challenges arise, we are programmed to take action, to jump in with both feet, and then to cope with the situations. The human mind is very good at solving problems, and we get great satisfaction from this ability. Without goals to attain and problems to solve, we quickly become frustrated and bored.

Michelangelo died in 1564 at the age of eighty-eight at a time when the life expectancy was about thirty-five. He was a vital, energetic man who went to sleep every night eager to wake up refreshed in the morning, ready to solve another problem. For Michelangelo, the painting, the sculpture, the solution already existed. Once he could push away the unnecessary confusion, he would find the answer waiting. He said that inside every piece of marble there was a sculpture, and all he had to do was chip away the excess marble—the statue would be there. What an extraordinary and powerful thought.

We are not perfect—far from it. Compared to a dog's sense of smell, ours is barely adequate. We can't run as fast as most animals, we certainly aren't as strong as a horse or an elephant, and a bird's eyes are many times sharper than ours. And yet we do pretty well, don't we? The reason is simple: In this time and place, and with the assets we have, we are *programmed for success.* Let's not stand in our own way.

Change Your
Response to Stress

Maybe you can't change all the little disturbances of life, but you can change your *responses* to them. And if you are to remain happy and healthy, you must understand that *you are in control.* Remember: You are not a victim, so don't act like a victim. Take charge. Change what needs to be changed.

This ability to change—to adapt—for our own good has been with us since human life on earth began. As noted earlier, Hans Selye considered adaptability to be "probably the most distinctive characteristic of life." I agree.

The first living things on earth faced a hostile and unforgiving environment. But living things persisted because they could do what rocks and other nonliving things could not do—they could *adapt* to their environment. The environment could not be changed to suit the first plants or animals, so the plants and animals changed to suit the environment, or they died. That is the essence of evolution.

Your ability to change is your greatest asset. Without it you would not be able to lead a decent life. *With it* you can be whatever you want to be. The ancient Greek scholar Epictetus said, "People are disturbed not by the things that happen, but by their *opinion* of the things that happen." So adapt and take charge of your responses.

Begin at the Beginning

When I have a patient who seems overwhelmed by life's challenges, we spend as much time discussing ways to dissipate that stress naturally as we spend going through purely medical procedures. Your mind and body are a team that makes up the whole person, and one team member affects the other. If you are feeling overwhelmed, your body often reacts, taking its cue from your mental state, and you become physically ill. However, this also works in reverse: a positive, uplifting mental outlook can give your body a jump-start on feeling well. But you can't do everything at once.

I find the best way to combat feeling overwhelmed by too many responsibilities is to think about one thing at a time and then concentrate on changing or adjusting one thing that will make you feel better for a week. That's what I would ask you to do if you came to my office. And you wouldn't leave until you had established that one goal for the week. It might be trying some kind of relaxation program, making a dietary change, getting into an exercise program, or simply finding some time for yourself in a busy schedule. When you are successful with changing that one element, you will be ready to accommodate another, and you will want to continue your changes.

In this case, I say, "Let's think about this week. What can you do to help yourself this week? Next week will follow. And so will the one after that. Don't try to do a hundred things at once. Take one thing at a time, even if you alone can't decide which thing is most important." I can help you; just *start with one thing.*

"A journey of a thousand miles begins with a single step," said Lao-tzu, the sixth-century B.C. Chinese philosopher who founded Taoism.

16

Establish a Good Relationship with Your Doctor

Our minds and bodies are inextricably tied together. Our mental state affects our physical state, and vice versa. One of the most effective healing tools we have is our own mind.

Sometimes the clue to illness can be found in a person's mental outlook. As I said before, I spend as much time talking with and listening to my patients as I do performing strictly medical procedures. I believe that a doctor must take a very detailed medical history from a patient to establish a solid doctor-patient relationship. The patient often inadvertently diagnoses a problem in the course of giving me his or her medical history. It is crucial for the physician to know how the patient views himself or herself in life and what kind of support system he or she has. You and your doctor must listen to each other.

17

Take Steps to Help Prevent Cancer

We can probably help prevent at least 85 percent of all cancers; the rest occur through abnormal changes (mutations) in cells, or through heredity. The number-one killer, lung cancer (which is caused largely by cigarette smoking), and the highly publicized industrial cancers, such as those that develop in people who work in chemical-related jobs or who are exposed to chemical wastes, are preventable. Many other cancers are preventable, too.

I believe—and many cancer experts agree—that many cancers are linked to an improper diet. If an improper diet can cause some cancers, it stands to reason that a proper diet can help prevent those cancers. For example, it is estimated that one-third of deaths due to cancer of the large intestine (colon) and rectum are preventable. Most cancers are preventable if we start thinking about prevention early enough.

Perhaps we have less control than we would like over the air we breathe, but we can control enough things in our lives to make a difference. For instance, how many of us take control when we order a meal in a restaurant? Too many people go into a restaurant, order a meal, and take what they get. The next time you go to a Chinese restaurant, for instance, try asking for the fish *without* the soy sauce, salt, and monosodium glutamate (MSG), and make sure you sit in the nonsmoking section. Also, think about your children, since many of the cancers that strike in middle age have their roots in poor childhood diets that could have been improved or in exposure to second-hand smoke from cigarettes.

No matter how hard we try to prevent cancer through a proper diet, we reduce our chances for success if we are under stress. Stress breaks down the body's immune system and allows malignant cancers to form that would have been deterred otherwise. My philosophy has always been that preventing a disease is preferable to treating it. Remember that an enjoyable physical activity like walking is great for reducing stress.

Think of your ability to prevent cancer in the same way that you prevent serious injuries or even death by using seat belts in your car. Once you realize that you *can* have some control over cancer, you will feel good about yourself by doing what you can to prevent it.

Many foods have built-in properties that help reduce the risk of cancer. For example, some excellent anticancer foods are bran, broccoli, brussels sprouts, carrots, citrus fruits, kale, pinto beans, skim-milk products, spinach, and sweet potatoes. Have you ever thought about eating a small, baked sweet potato as an afternoon snack?

Here are a few examples of the specific anticancer substances that some foods contain. Broccoli contains at least four substances that have anticancer properties: *sulforaphane,* a chemical that raises the activity of enzymes that counter the effects of carcinogens; *beta-carotene; vitamin C;* and *indoles* (nitrogen compounds). Sulforaphane is also found in brussels sprouts, cauliflower, kale, carrots, and green onions. Celery contains *3-n-butylphthalide,* which may lower blood pressure and blood cholesterol.

Bran is an excellent anticancer food, since its insoluble fiber reduces the risk of colon, prostate, and breast cancer. Wheat germ is one concentrated source of wheat bran. Wheat germ provides more protein than wheat bran, but wheat bran provides provides 12 grams of fiber per serving—the same as in eight pieces of whole-wheat bread. Processed bran or wheat germ can be sprinkled over cereals or other foods, and bran is also available in a handy capsule form. I usually take mine in the morning, but see what time of the day works best for you.

Strawberries are high in fruit fiber (pectin), which reduces cholesterol levels and the risk of hypertension, and may help prevent colon cancer. One-half cup of strawberries provides more fiber than a slice of whole-wheat bread.

Onions and garlic help lower blood pressure, reduce dangerous blood clotting, and lower "bad" cholesterol while raising the level of "good" cholesterol. They may also help prevent some cancers. Onions, which are rich in vitamin C, may inhibit the formation of tumors and lessen the effects of bronchial asthma. Garlic contains an "antibiotic" and decongestant compound, and it has been shown to boost immunity. (I talk more later about garlic's great properties.)

Recent research has underscored the benefits of using foods, rather than vitamin supplements, to help prevent cancer. Research has also indicated that a daily diet rich in fresh fruits and vegetables can help us maintain good health at all stages of life, and perhaps slow the progression of chronic diseases in our later years as well.

I recommend that you average three servings of fresh fruits and three servings of vegetables a day. Some foods to avoid are aged cheeses, animal fats, butter, cured meats, fried foods, low-fiber cereals and other low-fiber foods, smoked meats, and whole-milk products.

Eat More Fiber

A high-fiber diet lowers the risk of cancer of the large intestine. The fiber in foods such as bran, whole grains, leafy vegetables, and raw fruit with skin absorbs lots of moisture and adds bulk to your food as it passes through your intestines. As a result, your stool is larger, you have more frequent bowel movements, and you speed up the passage of feces through your large intestine.

The typical high-fat, high-sugar, low-fiber American diet causes constipation and allows feces to accumulate in the large intestine. The longer the feces remain there, the longer the noxious products in them will irritate the intestinal walls. A high-fiber diet speeds up the transit time of feces through the intestine, and thereby reduces the risk of colon cancer.

Ordinarily, low-fiber food is eliminated two or three days after it is eaten. With a high-fiber diet, however, the food is digested in 12 to 18 hours and usually is eliminated within 24 hours.

Eat a Low-Fat Diet to Lower Your Cancer Risks

The more researchers understand about the ingredients found in fruits, vegetables, beans, and herbs, the more impressed they are with the power of those ingredients to retard the cellular breakdown in the body that leads to cancer and other diseases. People who eat a plant-rich diet have lower rates of cancer than people who eat meat-rich diets.

There's no question anymore that we should be eating less fat, and most food producers are jumping on the bandwagon. I saw a label the other day that had in bold letters: "Low-Fat! Great Taste!" It was on a box of dog biscuits. Even our pets are reaping the benefits of low-fat eating. In fact, some pets have a healthier diet than their owners.

I recommend a low-fat, low-cholesterol diet. Your daily food intake should contain no more than 20 percent fat, as I noted earlier. (I think the Federal Dietary Guideline of 30 percent is too high.)

High-cholesterol foods such as egg yolks, brains, kidneys, sweetbreads, dairy products, and animal fats, including lard. High-fat foods include fatty beef, fatty pork, lamb, frankfurters, cake frosting, pies, butter and margarine, mayonnaise, and cooking fats and oils.

Fish, chicken, and turkey (white meat) contain acceptable levels of cholesterol. Egg whites, vegetables, fruits, and whole grains, including whole-grain cereals, do not contain *any* choles-terol. Many foods contain practically no fat. A few of these are skim milk, most fruits and vegetables (including potatoes), light rye bread, and cooked rice and pasta.

Statistically, a high-fat, high-cholesterol diet seems to be asso-ciated with cancer, especially of the colon, breast, and prostate. A study at the National Institute of Public Health in Stockholm has shown that a low-fat diet may help women avoid a recurrence of breast cancer after surgery to remove a malignant breast tumor.

A word of caution about "low-fat" and "fat-free" desserts, such as cookies: People are eating more of these desserts than ever before, and as a result, they are gaining more weight than ever before. Two suggestions: (1) Check the calorie count in one serving. (2) Check if you are eating only one serving.

FAT CONTENT OF VARIOUS FOODS

Food	Average Serving	Fat (grams)
Ground beef, broiled	3 ounces	17
Oils, salad and cooking	1 tablespoon	14
Pie, apple	1 piece (¹/₈ pie)	13
Butter	1 tablespoon	12
Mayonnaise	1 tablespoon	11
Cheese, American	1 ounce	9
Liver, beef, fried	3 ounces	9
Bacon	2 slices	8
Milk, whole	1 cup	8
Potato chips	10 chips	8
Egg	1 large	6
Salmon, pink, canned	3 ounces	5
Pizza, cheese	1 piece (¹/₈ pizza)	4
Yogurt, low-fat, with added milk solids	1 cup	4
Fish sticks	1 stick	3
Bread, white, enriched	1 slice	1
Milk, skim	1 cup	0
Peas, frozen	¹/₂ cup	0

Source: U.S. Department of Agriculture

Take Action
to Live Positively

The Golden Rule is an exhortation to be *positive*. It doesn't say, "*Don't* do anything to others that you *don't* want them to do to you." It says instead, "*Do* unto others as you *would* have them do unto you." It's not enough to say you *didn't* do anything wrong. What did you *do* right?

If you were to take a reckoning of your life on December 31 of every year, you would need to ask yourself not "What have I *not* done?" but rather "What *have* I done?" The eighteenth-century British statesman and philosopher Edmund Burke said, "The only thing necessary for the triumph of evil is for good men to do nothing."

You are different from anyone else in the whole world, so *make a difference.* And get involved in life. Life is a visceral experience. Get your hands dirty.

Banish Boredom

I remember many a rainy weekend when our four children couldn't leave our apartment to ride bikes or play ball in the park. Were they bored? Maybe for a little while, until one of the children got the idea to build a fort out of the sofa cushions, or to sit in a closet talking and giggling with the others, or to try on grown-up clothing and put on a show. Children are wonderful. They instinctively know that the other side of boredom is creativity.

Don't you wish you still had that flair for making something out of nothing? Well, you probably do, but something is always getting in your way. The next time you have "nothing to do," do something just for the fun of it—the sort of thing you *used* to do before life became so serious.

Get in Touch with Your Body

There are many things our bodies do for us automatically, with no help from us. For example, we don't have to think about breathing—we just do it. We breathe when we're working, when we're playing, and even when we're asleep.

But here's something I would like you to think about: Once in a while during the day, especially when you're feeling like things are getting out of control, take charge of your breathing. Stop and take a few deep, slow breaths. Give your body a message to slow down. And while you're at it, enjoy the wonderful physical feeling of those deep, slow breaths. It's a treat we have forgotten about, the same way we have forgotten about *laughing out loud.* Get back in touch with your body.

23

Eat Lots of Complex Carbohydrates

For years we have been taught that some foods are fattening and should be avoided. Foods like pasta, bread, potatoes, rice, and popcorn have been given a bad name. The truth is, these foods are all complex carbohydrates, and they are *great* for you. By all means, do not avoid them—just the opposite. I *want* you to eat pasta as often as you like, as long as you use a meatless marinara sauce, a fresh vegetable sauce, or low-salt chicken broth with it. (See the recipes on pages 207, 208, and 203.)

It's not the pasta that puts on the pounds (unless you're eating huge portions). It's the high-calorie cheeses and sauces you put on pasta. The same is true for popcorn, potatoes, rice, couscous, and many other whole-grain complex carbohydrates. When you're in the mood for a potato, make it a baked or boiled potato, not french fries. And forget the sour cream or butter. Instead, for toppings try low-fat yogurt with chives, herbs and spices (including freshly ground black pepper), a homemade tomato sauce, or other low-fat sauces.

Carbohydrate foods such as whole-grain bread, pasta, rice, cereal, vegetables, and fruits help us stay thin by stimulating our metabolisms to burn higher. Excess dietary fat is easily converted into body fat; excess carbohydrate is not. Therefore, if you want to overindulge with little danger of gaining weight, eat more complex carbohydrates. Have extra pasta, but try to extend the original portion of sauce over the larger portion of pasta. Eventually, you might prefer less sauce.

Here are some important words from Sophia Loren about complex carbohydrates: "Everything you see I owe to spaghetti."

24

Be Proud of Eating Well

In January 1992, a four-day conference was held in Cambridge, Massachusetts, to examine the pros and cons of a typical Mediterranean diet. As I expected, the benefits of such a low-fat, high-complex-carbohydrate diet are now being recognized. The conference suggested that our dietary intake of fat can slightly exceed 30 percent if we use unsaturated and polyunsaturated oils such as olive or canola oils.

But for some people there's a hitch to eating a high-complex-carbohydrate diet instead of a high-fat diet that includes frequent meals of beef and other red meats. The kinds of meals I described earlier—based on pasta, rice, beans, and vegetables—represent an unfavorable memory of poverty to many people. To these people, a fatty steak means affluence—a far step up from the childhood poverty they would like to forget.

My coauthor is Italian, and he remembers many meatless meals during his childhood in New York City. "The foods I remember most," he says, "are things like bread, pasta, beans, rice, olive oil, potatoes, tomatoes, melon, and lots of other fresh fruits and vegetables. Plenty of nights we had pasta *and* beans or potatoes or peas as a meal, or beans, rice, celery, and small pieces of bread." He also remembers spinach sandwiches, broccoli sandwiches, and even banana sandwiches. Both his parents are still alive, at ninety-three and eighty-five, with no signs of cancer or cardiovascular disease. Their diet remains basically the same.

Maybe our parents and grandparents ate a high-complex-carbohydrate diet because that's what they had available, but it turns out they were better off than the wealthiest people who ate a constant diet of sugar, salt, and fat and then died in their thirties or forties. We know much more about good eating than our ancestors did. Why not take advantage of that knowledge instead of looking for excuses to eat the "modern" way?

25

Be Your Own Tranquilizer

If you have ever taken a tranquilizer, you know that you were better able to cope with the petty annoyances that seemed so large before you took the medicine. The telephones didn't stop ringing; they just didn't bother you anymore. Your *response* to the outside world changed. Of course, nothing changed except the way you perceived and reacted to the outside stimuli. (Remember Epictetus; what he said will always come in handy, especially when you are least in the mood to be reminded of it: "People are disturbed not by the things that happen, but by their *opinion* of the things that happen.")

I prescribe tranquilizers, usually for short periods to help my patient change a pattern of behavior. But the thing I am really interested in is getting my patients to understand how they can be their *own* tranquilizers. They can learn not only to tell the difference between trivial and important things but also to stop reacting to *everything.*

One of the best natural tranquilizers is the low-impact exercise of walking. The first thirty minutes of a walk are for your body, but the rest, the best, are for your spirit. Walk at a comfortable pace for at least forty-five minutes to an hour, and the brain chemicals known as endorphins will kick into your system, providing a natural high.

26

Try Meditation

When we hear the word *meditation,* many of us think of a yogi sitting in the lotus position, deep in concentration, softly chanting. But there are many forms of meditation. For instance, if I have free time between patients' visits, I often sit quietly in my office chair, breathing deeply, with as little conscious thought as possible. I certainly am not in a trance or a mystical never-never land, but usually I can successfully block out the sounds of sirens and other street noises that are so much a part of every city. And how pleasant it is to be "on vacation" for fifteen or twenty minutes. How refreshing and reassuring it is to know that such an accessible respite is possible!

Controlled breathing is an important part of meditation. One of the aims of meditation is to gain some control of your unconscious mind. This is where deep, rhythmic breathing comes in. As you take control of your breathing (which you usually don't have to think about), you are establishing a connection between the conscious and unconscious parts of your mind. Breathing can be used the way some people repeat a *mantra,* or particular sound used in meditation.

When you meditate, remember these hints:

1. Sit comfortably, but not in a position that would cause you to fall asleep. Close your eyes. Take deep, regular breaths, and be

aware of taking the breaths. Think of one part of your body (such as your chest) that responds to your deep breathing.

2. Allow your breath to come and go without force or effort.

3. Do not become critical of yourself if your thoughts intrude. If your mind wanders, acknowledge that, and then gently escort yourself back to your breath—back to the present.

4. Experience what you are doing now. There is nothing "next." One definition of meditation is "Paying attention on purpose in the present."

Remember that relaxation is always available and that relaxation means being comfortable with yourself. Get used to setting aside a definite time each day for meditation, because special times need to be *ritualized.* A ritual honors a space in time.

27

Change What You Can, Accept What You Can't

Patients come into my office all the time just to talk. Nothing physical is wrong with them—they know that, even if they won't come right out and say it—but *something* is making them feel awful. Very often, after we've talked a while (or they've talked and I've listened), the patients make their own diagnoses—and they're often right.

Usually, what people have to do to feel better is to make some sort of change in their lives, even a small one. But the idea of making that change is scaring them and creating yet another problem.

Too many of us don't realize that sometimes we *can* change something in our lives that would make a difference. Instead, we go on *wishing* that something would happen to make us feel better. Have the courage to change the things you can, one at a time. You'll feel wonderful for doing it.

Reshape Your Eating Habits

A very interesting study was completed in 1992 that shows how eating habits can be changed for the better. On board the USS *Scott*, a naval destroyer, the 380 crew members were not given their regular menu during a six-month tour of duty. Instead, they were given a menu that adhered to the American Cancer Society's guidelines. For example, a traditional breakfast of hot buttered oatmeal, grilled or hard-boiled eggs, home-fried potatoes, bacon, and hot biscuits was replaced by fruit and assorted cold cereals with low-fat milk. Lunch and dinner items such as fried chicken, brown gravy, and buttered carrots were omitted, but plenty of tuna sandwiches, salad bars, and fruit were available. Cooking butter was replaced with a fat-free substitute.

As expected, most of the crew lost weight and reduced their cholesterol levels. What was not expected was that most of the crew members not only enjoyed the change, but decided to continue their new eating habits while on shore duty.

If 380 sailors who were used to being overfed can make this kind of a change, can't you? Of course you can, and you will have even more choices than they did. Keep reading, and you'll find lots of ways to change your eating habits without giving up all the good things in life. But most of all, remember that you *can* change the way you eat—and enjoy doing it!

29 ◇ Keep the Portions Sensible

Despite what your mother said, you do not have to eat everything on your plate, especially in a restaurant that serves overly generous portions.

When eating at home, remember to serve small to moderate portions. Then, eat slowly to give your stomach a chance to register that it is full, and to signal your brain with that information. It makes much more sense to finish small portions than to waste (or eat) excessive portions.

Walk, Walk, Walk

There is no doubt in my mind that walking is the best physical activity, for lots of reasons. You don't have to be an athlete to walk, you don't have to learn how to do it, you don't need a pool or gym or tennis court, you can do it alone or with a friend (including your dog), you don't need a special outfit, and you don't even have to take a shower afterward. Walking is safe for just about everybody, and it's free. It also burns fat.

Among other things, walking helps prevent constipation, varicose veins, tension, and high blood pressure. It tones your muscles, relieves stress, improves your circulation, and helps you lose weight. Other physical activities may achieve the same results; walking is by no means the only physical activity you can or should do. But for my money it is the *best,* and it may also be the only activity you *will* do—which is one of its biggest advantages. Good food is not good if you don't eat it, and a good physical activity is not good if you don't do it. We all walk, and that automatically makes walking a good physical activity. Just do it! And do *more* of it.

No less an authority than the ancient Greek physician Hippocrates, the father of medicine, claimed that "walking is man's best medicine."

Use Your Head

When I asked one of my overweight patients why she kept eating sweet junk food, she told me that when things were difficult—stressful at home or at work—the only sweetness she had in her life was ice cream and cookies. The sweet food became a substitute for the sweetness she did not find in her life.

I saw her point, and I told her so. I marveled at her honest self-analysis. She knew why she was doing something unhealthy, but I wanted her to understand why she had chosen unwisely. After listening to her very carefully, I was able to point out that she already knew how to initiate a plan to stop her unhealthy pattern. She agreed, and went on to say that she would expand the idea of "sweetness" to include the good feeling brought on by a long walk, a bike ride, dancing, or lunch with a friend. "Sweetness" could be a *positive* thing. And it worked!

As I've said before, I've often found that patients have the ability to diagnose their own problems. And when they are part of discovering the solution, they are better able to maintain the necessary willpower and interest to make permanent changes in their lifestyles.

32

Look Squarely at Your Eating Habits

We Americans are now consuming less palm and coconut oil (both very fatty), whole milk, beef, and butter than we did in the past. That sounds good, but listen to some other statistics: We are eating 40 percent more cheese, cream, sour cream, and high-fat dips. And we are consuming over 50 percent more high-salt snacks. Although we are eating more chicken, most of it is *fried.* We are eating more sugar, high-fat ice cream, and hamburgers, and restaurant portions are continuing to get larger. (Nobody seems to be complaining about the overwhelming size of restaurant portions, but you should be.)

Believe me, our eating habits only *seem* to be getting better. We're talking more about health, but we're eating more of many unhealthy foods. (We are eating huge portions of "low-fat" foods, to the point where they have become a major source of weight gain.)

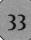

Be Physically Active to Help Prevent Cardiovascular Disease

Your heart is the most important muscle in your body—don't neglect it. Physical activity helps your heart work at peak efficiency, and it helps keep your blood pressure under control by reducing the buildup of cholesterol and plaque on the inner walls of your blood vessels. By strengthening your heart and your entire cardiovascular system, physical activity will definitely reduce your chances of developing cardiovascular disease.

In July 1992, the American Heart Association classified insufficient physical activity as a "risk factor" for cardiovascular disease, ranking it along with high blood pressure, high blood cholesterol, and smoking. Previously, a sedentary lifestyle had been classified as the less serious "contributing factor."

Walking is the healthiest, safest aerobic exercise. It will lower your blood pressure, relieve stress, help you think more clearly, reduce body fat, and strengthen your cardiovascular system. For the best cardiovascular benefits, you need to exercise at the proper intensity for at least forty-five minutes at a time. To find the proper intensity, or your target heart rate, subtract your age from 220; the result is a maximum figure. Plan to exercise between 70 and 80 percent of this maximum. For example, let's assume you are a forty-five-year-old woman: 220-45=175, then 70 percent of 175 is 122, and 80 percent of 175 is 140.

So to improve your cardiovascular system, you should exercise at an intensity that produces a pulse rate of 122 to 140 beats per minute. The easiest place on your body to find your pulse is probably on your throat, just below your jaw and next to your Adam's apple. Press gently so you don't interrupt the flow of blood and produce an inaccurate reading. Also, use your fingers, not your thumb, since your thumb may have a beat of its own that throws you off. Find your pulse rate for ten seconds, and then multiply that number by six to get the number of beats per minute.

34 Be Consistent

A steady program of moderate physical activity (such as brisk walking) will do you more good than a year of vigorous exercise followed by a lapse into inactivity. You owe it to your body to establish a lifestyle it can get used to and rely on. "Yo-yo" dieting and on-again, off-again exercise programs can actually do more harm than good because they disrupt your body's natural rhythms.

Just the way you can confuse your children or co-workers by telling them something one day and then contradicting it the next, so you can also confuse your body, putting unnecessary stress on it by changing the rules over and over again. Your body is geared to maintain a consistency even when things outside your body are changing. Go along with the idea of consistency when it comes to good eating habits and regular physical activity. Let your body relax into a steady, healthy routine.

Walk Wisely

I believe that walking is the best all-around "exercise." Try it and see if you don't agree.

1. Start walking about a mile a day and gradually increase the distance. Try to walk at least 3 or 4 miles every day. (That's not as much as you think it is, especially if you follow an interesting route.) If you can't do 3 or 4 miles daily, walk at least three times a week, with a minimum of 2.5 miles a day.

2. Breathe deeply, swing your arms, keep your body erect and your head up, pull in your abdomen, and walk as briskly as you can. If you lean forward at the waist, you may hurt your back and make breathing difficult.

3. Stretch your muscles and warm up slowly before starting to walk. Cool down by walking slowly when you are through. Select a pleasant route that is as level as possible. You can tackle the hills and inclines a little later, when you're in better shape. Summertime walking is best done in the shade, at least for part of the way. Vary your routes so you don't get bored. (If you walk in the road, always walk against the traffic so you can see what's coming.) For a change of pace use a running track once a week if it is available.

4. You do not have to spend $150 for a walking suit. Put your money into good walking shoes or sneakers, and dress comfort-

ably. Don't overdress in the summer; heavy sweating will not help you lose weight, but it could cause heat exhaustion. Loose-fitting cotton clothes are recommended, including cotton socks, because they allow sweat to escape. (Woolen socks are not recommended.) Get a good pair of walking socks in a sporting goods store. In very cold weather add layers of light clothing, and wear a hat or hood to keep body heat from escaping.

5. Walking in the rain and at night requires your special attention. If you walk in the rain, you'll be more comfortable with waterproof clothes. At night carry a flashlight and wear white or yellow clothes, or clothes with reflective surfaces so that drivers can see you on the road. Don't take it for granted that drivers will see you— keep to the side of the road.

6. Take a drink of water before you walk, and drink as much as you want afterward. Water is very important to your body.

7. Walk at any time of the day that suits you, but in the summer you'll probably be happier in the morning or early evening, when there is relief from the sun. Also, taking a walk before dinner is a great way to decrease your appetite at the time of day when you should eat the least.

8. If you carry a tote bag when you walk during working hours in the city, or to and from work, carry the bag across your body, with the strap on your shoulder and the bag on the opposite hip. If all the weight is on one side of your body, your spine could start to curve irregularly. Switch shoulders occasionally.

9. If you have an injury, don't try to walk until it heals. If you feel a strain that could lead to an injury, slow down or stop. Be especially careful when walking downhill or up slopes. Both situations can throw you off balance, and they cause an abnormal strain on your feet, ankles, legs, and hips.

10. If you live in the city, walk instead of taking a bus or a taxi. If you must take a bus or a taxi, get off ten blocks early and walk the rest of the way. If you are waiting for a bus, start walking toward your destination until the bus comes. Most city dwellers have little trouble finding interesting routes.

11. Many people have become serious "mall walkers." At least one major athletic shoe company has developed a walking shoe for use on the hard, slick surfaces of indoor shopping malls.

12. Don't think of walking as a "workout" or boring exercise. Make it fun. Select a safe and lovely route, and enjoy yourself!

Brisk walking is preferred, but any pace is better than none at all. In fact, according to the authors of a 1991 study published in the *Journal of the American Medical Association,* women who walk three miles a day, five days a week, reduce their risk of heart disease. Walking, no matter what the pace, increases high-density lipoproteins (HDLs, the "good" cholesterol) in the blood. The study also found that brisk walking can be as beneficial as jogging for increasing cardiovascular fitness.

About seventy million Americans are being treated for cardio-vascular disease, and many others have it and don't know it. Walking improves the circulation of the blood and relieves your heart from doing too much work. Your heart is a pump, and it works hard all the time, beating about 100,000 times a day, and pumping and repumping about 72,000 quarts of blood throughout your body each day. As remarkable as your heart is, it can still use all the help it can get. Walking is a wonderful solution.

Walk for 45 minutes to an hour. To find out how far you are walking, measure a mile by driving it in your car, or by walking with a pedometer. Then time yourself while walking that mile. If it takes you 25 minutes, you are walking at a pace of 2.4 miles per hour. When you can walk comfortably for 45 to 60 minutes, increase your pace so that you walk farther in that time. For an overweight person, 3 miles per hour is a fast walking pace. For a person in generally good health, anything under 3 miles per hour is slow. Normally, 3.5 to 4.5 miles per hour is the optimum brisk pace, but work up to it slowly.

Don't Count Calories

For every 100 calories consumed from carbohydrates, your body uses 23 to convert the food into body fat. This leaves only 77 carbohydrate calories to be stored as fat. But your body treats the fat in your diet differently. For every 100 calories of dietary fat, your body uses only 3 calories in the conversion process. This leaves 97 calories to be stored as fat in your body. So it stands to reason that with a high-complex-carbohydrate diet your body does not accumulate fat. But with a high-fat diet, the pounds and the inches pile on.

You can see that it is much smarter to eat 100 calories of complex carbohydrates rather than 100 calories of fat. That's one of the reasons I don't want you to count calories—it's *where* those calories come from that matters. Eat moderate amounts of foods high in complex carbohydrates and low in fat, and you will be healthy and trim.

The simple truth of weight loss is this: Eat less fat than you are burning off each day, and you will lose weight. And a high-complex-carbohydrate diet will give you more energy.

Eat a Healthy Amount of Fat

Unfortunately, some people think that if a *low*-fat diet is good, a *no*-fat diet is even better. But the truth is, a *no*-fat diet is dangerous to your health. So is a *no*-salt diet or a *no*-sugar diet. The key word is *low,* not *no.*

Please do not try to eliminate *all* fat from your diet. Fat is an essential part of your diet, but you don't need much of it. In fact, words like *all, no, never,* and *always* rarely fit into a sensible, balanced lifestyle.

Of the three types of fatty acids—saturated, monounsaturated, and polyunsaturated—only polyunsaturated fats are considered essential in the diet because our bodies cannot manufacture them. In other words, to get a healthy supply of polyunsaturated fats, we must eat foods that contain them. Such foods include vegetable oils, seeds, nuts, and green vegetables such as broccoli. Monounsaturated fats are even more beneficial than polyunsaturated fats.

If the body is not supplied with enough polyunsaturated fat, it will begin to use the other types of fatty acids instead. Eventually, this lack of polyunsaturated fat can lead to hardening of the arteries. *But,* don't start overdosing on polyunsaturated fats. As usual, too much is just as bad as too little.

Try a Vegetarian Fare

Vegetarians who eat a balanced diet seem to have fewer ill-nesses than nonvegetarians. Also, most vegetarians live longer. One of the reasons for this good fortune is that vegetarian diets are generally low in fat (about as low as I'd like *your* diet to be—no more than 20 percent of your total calories).

I suggest to my patients that they work toward having meatless dinners three or four times a week. Let a few ounces of poultry or fish be supplements to your main vegetable or whole-grain dish. An easy way to accomplish such a goal is to prepare vegetable stir-fries with a few ounces of meat. Being a partial vegetarian by eating meat-less meals a few days a week is an excellent and healthy lifestyle.

One of the greatest fears of people who are thinking about becoming vegetarians is that they won't get enough protein. This was a bigger problem in the past than it is now, when we know so much about nutrition. Discuss it with your physician, and you will see how easy it is to get protein from beans, lentils and other legumes, tofu, and whole-grain foods (including wheat germ). You will get all the other nutrients you need from vegetables and the rest of your diet, without the extra calories in sugar and fat. Check with your physician to make sure you are not tending toward defi-ciencies of vitamin B12 and iron, and have your blood count checked to detect a low level of iron.

Incidentally, if you decide to eat everything but meat, fish, and poultry, you are a *lacto-ovovegetarian*. Vegetarians who eat no animal products, including milk and eggs, are *vegans*. Those who eat dairy products but not eggs are *lactovegetarians*.

My personal recommendation is that you include fish in your vegetarian diet. Fish contains omega-3 fatty acids, which are good. Other animal fats contain omega-6 fatty acids, which are neutral. Do not eat raw fish, which can contain harmful parasites and can cause stomach cancer. (Stomach cancer is fairly common in Japan, where eating raw fish is the norm.)

39

Get Beyond
"Inherited" Fatness

I have patients who say, "I never had a chance. Both my parents are fat, my grandparents were fat, all of my brothers and sisters are fat, even my dog is fat. I guess I just have to get used to being fat too." Actually, we're still not sure exactly how much genetics counts toward being fat. What we *do* know is that a fat child frequently grows up to be a fat adult.

On the surface it would appear that fatness is inherited, because when both parents are fat, they usually have fat children. But environmental influences are very strong and could easily contribute to family fatness. Very often, fat parents feed their children too much food from the time the children are born. If children are taught to overeat while they are very young, they probably will grow up to overeat as adults. Of course, that pattern can be changed. You don't have to accept being overweight as a way of life. A change is possible, and I have seen it happen many times.

It is thought that a child's pattern of fat cells develops during the crucial first two years of life. Overeating causes the number of fat cells to increase. Once fat cells become overabundant through a pattern of overeating, the *number* of cells always remains higher than normal, but the *size* of the cells can change. In other words, if you now have "fat" fat cells, you can someday have "skinny" fat cells.

Although obesity itself may not be a totally inherited factor, the *potential* to be fat probably *is* inherited. However, a child who has the potential to be fat does not necessarily have to *be* fat. If a child is physically active and eats the proper foods in the proper amounts—that is, does not overeat—the chances are good that he or she will remain lean. In contrast, a child raised in a family environment where too much food is eaten and there is too little (if any) physical activity will probably become overweight.

Eat More Mini-meals

People who eat on the run tend to get into the habit of eating several mini-meals during the day, and this style may carry over into nighttime, when they are at home. My inclination is not to fight a person's natural rhythm, as long as that person is benefiting from it.

Eating several *small* meals during the day is usually an excellent way of keeping your energy level high, while giving your body a chance to burn off separate, small packets of calories. If you prefer to eat that way, go ahead, but remember that for eating on the run and eating several mini-meals a day to be healthy, you should keep to fresh fruits or vegetables and grains—complex carbohydrates. Also remember that mini *means* mini.

One large daily meal is more fattening than three or four small ones. When you eat a large meal, your body responds by secreting more digestive juices, and you digest the food faster. As a result, you become hungry soon after the meal. (This may be the reason why we become hungry soon after a Chinese meal, which we usually consume quickly and in large quantities.) Also, it is easier and healthier to digest small meals, and your body needs nourishment more than once a day.

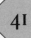

Cut the Sugars
to Help Your Heart

My eating plan is low in simple sugars for one obvious reason: simple sugars are fattening. But there are other reasons as well. A low amount of simple sugars in your diet decreases fatty acids in your blood and lessens the risk of a heart attack.

The average American eats more than 100 pounds of simple sugar a year. That's a lot of sugar. Just about every processed food contains sugar, usually more than we would guess—the amounts are not always printed on the labels. Incidentally, even though I feel strongly that sugar is not good for you, I would prefer that you use a *small amount* of sugar (or none at all) in your coffee or tea rather than artificial sweeteners, which may be carcinogenic.

When you eat simple sugar you cause an increase of fatty acids, or triglycerides, in your blood. Triglycerides combine with your normal blood glycerol to form the same kinds of fat as animal fat—the *same fats* that you have been told repeatedly to avoid.

I once had a patient who, when she first consulted me, had one of the highest triglyceride levels I had ever seen. It was 762, compared to the recommended level of 100 to 140! When she started eating according to my plan, this woman weighed 220 pounds. Within four months she lost 40 pounds and her triglyceride level dropped to 354. Two months later she was still losing weight, and her triglyceride level was normal.

Extra weight—even 15 to 20 percent—will probably increase your risk of developing some form of cardiovascular disease, especially if you are over forty years old. If you are overweight, you almost double your chances of dying from a heart attack. The fatter you are, the worse off you are.

Recognize Different Sugars

I want you to eat fresh fruit every day, but like everything else, in moderation. It's important to remember that fruit contains sugar in the form of fructose. Fructose is just another form of regular sugar, with the same characteristics that sugar has, although the sugar in fruit is less concentrated than in foods that contain simple sugar. The real point is, eat fruit in moderation, not ten portions a day. Three is enough.

Don't snack on fruit unless you can be satisfied with one piece at a time. I have a patient who works at home. He used to eat several pieces of fruit for breakfast, snack on dried fruit between meals, and often have fruit for lunch. He couldn't understand why he was tired all the time. In fact, he was usually so tired by dinnertime that he didn't want dinner (although he did manage some fruit). Not only is such a diet dangerous because it is so unbalanced, but it also contains a lot of sugar, and sugar makes you tired.

You shouldn't believe the ads that say that a candy bar will give you the energy you need to get through the long afternoon. A candy bar will pick you up for a very short time, and then will drop you—hard.

The guidelines from the federal government suggest three to five servings of fresh fruit each day, but as I said before, I think three are enough. Check the "breakfast" drinks starting on page 132 for another delicious way to consume fruit.

43 ◆ Make Stress Less Stressful

The late Hans Selye, probably the leading expert on stress, defined *stress* as "the nonspecific response of the body to any demand made upon it." Stress can be anything from losing your job to crying with excitement or pleasure. It doesn't matter whether the source of stress is pleasant or unpleasant. Both types of stress demand that your body adjust to a change in the environment.

Stress is a normal, sometimes unavoidable part of life. No matter how hard we try to change it, there will always be traffic jams during rush hour, and rain will always be wet. We can't change those simple facts. When we forget that some stressful situations are normal, we tend to overreact to them.

Another source of troublesome stress comes from unpleasant situations that we *should* try to change. For example, do you have a job that is, and always will be, frustrating and unrewarding? Do your windshield wipers smear instead of wipe? Does your clock never show the correct time? Is your reading light too dim? Is your reading light too bright? *Those* things should not be a source of stress for you. You can change every one of them.

If it needs fixing, fix it. If it *really* can't be changed, learn to accept it graciously and maturely. Both of those last words are important: graciously and maturely. Don't whine about something you can't possibly change—accept it graciously.

Make two lists:

(1) Things I can change and (2) Things I cannot change. When you're certain that you've been honest on both lists, do something about the items in the first list, and then learn to make the best of the items in the second list.

44 ◆ Be Open to Change

Recently I bumped into a friend whom I hadn't seen for a few years. The last time I had seen Anna, she was suffering from a rare form of autoimmune rheumatoid arthritis that was threatening to cripple her, although she was only forty-five years old.

At that time, the disease was beginning to disfigure her hands, and she had developed patches of an unidentified rash. She was taking large amounts of painkillers and experimental drugs, since her physicians had not made a complete diagnosis and were not sure how to treat her. They did warn her, however, that the quality of her life would be reduced, and that she would not be able to ski or do some other physical activities she enjoyed.

When I saw Anna the other day, five years after the onset of the disease, she looked happy and healthy. She had been through a round of chemotherapy and was still on daily medication, but she was as active as she wanted to be, and she had even gone skiing during the past winter.

"I'm driving my doctors crazy," she said. "I'm doing all the things they said I wouldn't be able to do."

This was fascinating, so I asked her what had happened since I had seen her last. She said she had been keeping a daily journal, recording how she reacted to medication, physical activity, food, rest, and so on. By tracking her progress so carefully, she was able to highlight cause-and-effect situations that her physicians may have missed. "I know my body very well," she said, "and I wouldn't do anything to hurt it."

As a result, she was able to make suggestions about medication and other parts of her treatment, and she was right more often that not. Naturally, her physicians were delighted (although puzzled). By working together, Anna and her physicians have been able to defeat Anna's potentially horrible disease as long as she remains on medication.

Anna was so positive about her happy ending that it rubbed off on the physicians. When she asked about her prospects, they told her that with so many advances in autoimmune research they should be able to turn her disease around completely in a few years.

I hope this happy, positive story of someone who truly minded her body can help you mind your own body more, too.

Slow Your Pace

Although most people who are overweight do not have hormonal problems, they may have some body differences that keep them overweight. For instance, overweight people frequently have a high level of insulin in their blood—most often caused by eating the wrong foods and overeating in general. The extra insulin encourages obesity by helping to convert sugar into fat quickly.

On top of this, the increased insulin may actually stimulate the appetite. Not only do fat people have more than the usual desire to eat, but the food they eat is converted into fat more rapidly.

You can overcome this problem. One way is to eat slowly. The faster you eat, the faster your insulin will act on sugar to turn it into fat.

The second way to combat this problem is to start a physical activity program such as walking. After a few weeks, your body will become more efficient at burning fat. The speed of your walking is not as important as its duration. The longer you walk, the more efficient your body is at burning fat in the fuel mix, and you will lose weight. If you are able to walk twice a day for forty-five minutes at a time, you will burn even more fat because your body will be in an almost constant state of higher metabolic activity.

Remember, just because you have a *tendency* to gain weight doesn't mean you *have to* gain weight.

Do the Physical Activities You Enjoy

The word *exercise* can be a problem for some people. But trust me: Exercise is not only good for your heart, your muscles, your senses, and your brain, but also wonderful for your self-esteem. If you think you don't like to exercise, just try walking or using a cross-country skiing machine or doing *something* else for a few weeks. And then listen to your body honestly. I have said it over and over: Our bodies were meant to move. We perform better when we move. It is what your body wants. Listen to it. And *do* it.

Forget the word *exercise*, and think instead of *physical activity* or simply *moving*. For some people, prescribed exercise, by its very nature, is boring, painful, and even expensive. You cannot be fit if you won't move. *Find one or two activities you like to do.*

Here are some other suggestions and facts that may give you some positive ideas about physical activity:

1. Don't fall into the trap of thinking of physical activity as an athletic event. Too many people, especially if they are overweight, don't want to play tennis or squash, or even run, because they are not natural athletes, or because they feel embarrassed about looking silly or losing the game, or both, so they end up staying home, doing nothing.

2. In this book I talk a lot about walking. I think it is the best all-around physical activity and the perfect solution to the whole "exercise problem." By walking vigorously for about forty-five minutes a day and eating sensibly, you could lose about fifteen unwanted pounds a year.

But first I want to mention a few other effective activities. Incidentally, nothing is ideal for everybody. Before you start any kind of physical activity program, you should check with your physician. Jumping rope is a great muscle toner and calorie burner, but it's not easy to jump rope without tripping all over yourself. So try jumping rope *without the rope.* If you make believe you're holding a rope, and move your arms as though you were, you will get toned up, and you won't have to worry about being intimidated by a rope. You'd be surprised how fancy and efficient you can get with a make-believe rope. Jump for only a minute or two to start with, but do it several times a day. Soon you will be able to jump for five minutes, then ten, and then longer. (Women should wear a supportive sports bra to help prevent tissue damage to their breasts.)

3. If you engage in a physical activity four or five times a week, you'll about triple the effectiveness of an activity done only three times a week. A physical activity done once or twice a week may have only a minimal effect.

4. Physical activity before meals *decreases* your appetite. Also, according to a study at Cornell University's Division of Nutritional Sciences, physical activity done about forty minutes *after* meals can help you burn off even more calories, and faster than usual.

5. One of the most sedentary activities is watching television. If you snack while you watch, you compound the problem immeasurably. If you are going to watch four hours of television every

night no matter what anyone tells you, at least try to do two things:

Don't eat traditional snack food while you watch television. If you must eat something, have some fresh fruit or vegetables. Most of us have been conditioned to stock up on things to eat and drink the minute we enter a movie theater. This conditioning carries over to our television watching. Eat a good dinner instead, and drink water or a cup of herb tea instead of snacking. You may also have a cup (not ten cups) of unbuttered, unsalted popcorn *or* a piece of fresh fruit *or* a drink you make in your blender with fresh fruit; see the recipes for blender drinks starting on page 133. Don't have all three snacks.

But what I really want you to do is break the after-dinner-snacking habit altogether, especially if you eat the full dinners I recommend.

The second thing I would like you to do is *get up from your chair at each commercial break and move around.* If your television set is downstairs, walk upstairs at a brisk pace and have a glass of water. If the set is upstairs, walk downstairs. If you don't have any stairs, get up and move around anyway. Some of my patients have stationary bikes or other equipment that they use during commercials or during athletic events when they don't have to hear every word the announcer is saying.

There are several reasons why people who watch a lot of television tend to gain weight: (1) They snack while they watch, (2) their sedentary style doesn't burn off calories, and (3) their metabolism is actually slowed down by the almost hypnotic effect of the programs.

6. If you lose weight through "dieting" alone, you will not look as fit as when you combine my positive eating suggestions with

physical activity. You don't want to lose weight and *still* look flabby. You want to lose weight and look lean and firm. Only physical activity will accomplish that.

7. When people tell me they are too tired to do any physical activity, I tell them they are putting the cart before the horse: if they were physically active, they wouldn't be so tired. (Some people think they are tired when they are really bored. The same people probably think they are hungry when they are really bored.) Be that as it may, very often our bodies do become tired because of a lack of activity. The only solution is to break the pattern by taking a walk, riding an exercise bike, using the stairs instead of the escalator, or doing any number of other physical activities. You will find out soon enough how quickly physical activity invigorates you. It will make your tiredness disappear.

Inactivity is one of your body's worst enemies. Your body was meant to be active. *How* you keep active is secondary, as long as your way is safe. Walk, dance, or just move around to a recording of some music that gets you moving. Move, move, move. If you keep moving, you will feel and look better for the rest of your life.

Drink Plenty of Water

Drink six to eight glasses of water a day to get the full benefit of a high-fiber diet. Water is good for you, and it encourages weight loss and weight maintenance. Some of my patients keep a special cup or recyclable eight-ounce plastic cups in the kitchen to remind them to drink water. The sight of the cups actually triggers the desire for water.

Just to show you how important water is, here's an interesting fact: We can live without food for weeks, but without water we would be dead in about three days. Did you know that the adult body is about 60 percent water, and that about 75 percent of the brain is water?

Don't wait until you feel thirsty to drink water, because thirst is not a reliable indicator of your body's need for water. Your body needs a steady supply of six to eight glasses of water a day, whether or not you feel thirsty. If you exercise heavily, you may need more than eight glasses. When you exercise, it is important to drink a glass of water fifteen to thirty minutes before you start. Drink as much water afterward as you need.

Rethink Your Favorite Meal

A Gallup Poll conducted in November 1991 showed that the typical American woman's ideal meal consisted of:

Shrimp cocktail or other seafood appetizer
Green salad
Vegetable soup
Steak
Potatoes and broccoli
Bread
Cheesecake or ice cream
Tea, hot or iced

I'm pleased to say that that's an excellent meal (as long as you avoid high-fat salad dressings and high-fat sauces), with two small changes: Try chicken or fish instead of steak, and sorbet or fresh fruit instead of cheesecake or ice cream.

Eat All Kinds of Foods

It is important to eat a well-balanced diet and to experiment with the taste of new foods. Your body was meant for a *variety* of foods.

One of the most harmful things that any "diet" can do is to remove foods that are needed for good health. Your diet must provide a well-balanced, nutritious selection of foods; otherwise, you are flirting with sickness. Many people on "high-something, low-everything-else" diets complain of being sluggish, irritable, and sexually impotent. Their skin and hair become dry and brittle, they become constipated because they are eating fewer high-fiber foods, blood cholesterol can go up, and malnutrition may become a reality.

I have a patient who used to eat only fried chicken, mashed potatoes, and sodas—*nothing* else. Talk about an unbalanced diet! He still eats plenty of chicken, but now it's baked or broiled instead of fried, and he even includes vegetables, pasta, and fish in his diet. He drinks water, iced tea, or fresh fruit juice and seltzer, instead of soda. After a while, his high blood pressure returned to normal, and he lost fifteen pounds. Still only in his mid-forties, he has understood that he has improved the quality and duration of his life immeasurably.

Eat all kinds of foods. Variety is what your body wants.

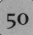

Enjoy Parties,
Vacations, and Holidays

Taking your healthy lifestyle on vacations can be even more challenging than going to a party. To be realistic, you probably should not expect to lose weight while you are on vacation. In fact, don't even try. If you have worked hard to acquire and live a healthy lifestyle, you deserve a break. Don't think about it consciously. Try to live naturally. You will probably burn off more calories than you think if you are sightseeing, walking, or swimming.

Vacations are important. They should be enjoyed as fully as possible, without the usual pressures and timetables. Relax and enjoy your vacation. In fact, vacation time is a good test to see how far you have come toward maintaining a healthy lifestyle. You may not even be tempted to eat improperly or to forget physical activity.

Know ahead of time that you will stray a bit, and don't feel guilty when it happens. Cut back a little on dinner if you have eaten a little too much during the day. Or walk an extra thirty minutes in the morning.

Vacations usually offer plenty of opportunities for physical activity. By all means relax in the lodge, but not all the time. If nothing else, walk and explore the new territory. An interesting phenomenon that has become more popular recently is the "fitness vacation." Besides playing tennis and golf, you can go cycling, horseback riding, rafting, kayaking, climbing, walking, skiing, or swimming, or do just about anything else you can think of.

Check with your physician before you plan a vigorous vacation. Please do not plan on doing more physical activity on your vacation than you would do otherwise, and make sure you have the proper clothing and equipment without overdoing it. It's a vacation, not a fashion show.

Have you ever made the mistake of declining a piece of cake at a birthday party? It's a sure way to look like a villain. Take the cake with a smile; you don't have to eat it all. There is so much going on at a party that you could easily put your plate down somewhere as you move off to check the presents or help pour the coffee or juice. There is no need to hurt your host's or hostess's feelings and call undue attention to yourself by making a fuss about food. Your host and hostess have worked all day (maybe even longer) to plan and prepare a party or dinner. It's a special occasion for them—don't spoil it.

51

Help Your Heart by Eating Food Fiber

Cardiovascular disease has been linked to diet even more than cancer has. In the United States, cardiovascular disease is responsible for more deaths than all other causes *combined.* In 1990, the last year for which figures are available, cardiovascular disease killed 930,477 people in the United States—43 percent of all U.S. deaths that year. In addition, it is estimated that over seventy million Americans have some form of cardiovascular disease, including high blood pressure.

During the past few decades the American diet has changed to include more animal protein, especially beef. Such a diet means a large increase in saturated fats and cholesterol, both of which have been implicated in cardiovascular diseases. If saturated fats and cholesterol are allowed to accumulate, they can stick to the inner walls of your arteries, narrowing the space for the passage of blood. Also, the elasticity of the arteries begins to disappear.

Such a condition is called *atherosclerosis.* It is dangerous because it cuts down blood flow, and if the artery is closed off entirely, no blood flows through at all. If the closed artery is in the heart, a heart attack occurs. If the artery takes blood to the brain, a stroke occurs.

52

Eat Less Fat

Fat is a killer. High-fat diets have been linked to cancer of the colon, rectum, breast, pancreas, and prostate gland. Reduce the amount of fat in your diet to 15 to 20 percent of the total weight of food you consume. Follow these guidelines:

Eat less of these foods:

1. *Fatty beef*—For the occasional times you want to eat beef, use the cuts that contain little internal fat (often these are the least expensive cuts), and remove all visible fat.

2. *Fatty lamb and veal*

3. *Pork and pork products*—Try to eat only lean pork, which is readily available.

4. *All fatty meats,* including sausages, cold cuts, and frank-furters

5. *Brazil, cashew, and macadamia nuts, and peanuts*

6. *Duck, goose, and other fatty fowl*

7. *High-fat cheese and other high-fat dairy products,* including whole milk

8. *Mayonnaise*—Low-fat mayonnaise is available. (Also, see the recipe on page 215 for blender mayonnaise, which contains no salt or saturated fat.)

9. *High-fat cakes and other pastries*

10. *Custards and puddings*

11. *Deep-fried foods*

12. *Animal cooking fats and oils,* including lard

Eat instead:

1. *Fish*

2. *Chicken and turkey,* mostly white meat, without skin

3. *Low-fat or skim milk; low-fat cheese, yogurt, and other dairy products—No-*fat frozen yogurt is available, but I personally prefer the taste of low-fat yogurt.

4. *Vegetable oil—*Preferably, use olive, canola, safflower, or corn oil, but any vegetable oil or a combination of vegetable oil and first-pressed, cold-pressed olive oil. (Cold-pressed olive oil contains a combination of monounsaturated and polyunsaturated fats that is beneficial.) Here is a quick rundown of oil types:

Oil	*Saturated Fat, by Percentage*
Canola	6
Safflower	10
Sunflower	11
Corn	13
Olive	14
Soybean	15
Peanut	18
Cottonseed	27
Palm	52
Coconut	92

5. *Beans and peas*

6. *Dry-roasted sunflower seeds*

7. *Pasta*

8. *Couscous*
9. *Rice*
10. *Potatoes*
11. *Whole-grain bread*
12. *Melon*

In addition to being implicated in some cancers, fat is also one of the two main causes of obesity; the other is underactivity. The core of a successful weight-management program is a menu high in complex carbohydrates and very low in fat. The best way to lose body fat is through physical activity, which uses body fat as its main source of energy. As I noted earlier, I recommend that no more than 20 percent of your total caloric intake be from fat, although the Federal Dietary Guidelines suggest 30 percent. Most Americans are eating at least twice as much fat as they should. (A low-fat diet is not advisable for babies. Check with your pediatrician to find out when your child is old enough for a regular low-fat diet.)

You can get charts from the U.S. Department of Agriculture that list food nutrients, and fat gram counters are also available at your bookstore. Also, I have listed the amount of fat in some foods in the tables on pages 172 to 177. But I would like to repeat an important point here: If you follow the basic principles of my plan, you will not have to count fat grams, at least not after a short period of getting used to the general amounts of fat in different foods.

Remember: It isn't the pasta or the potatoes or the bread that makes you fat. What goes *on* the pasta, potatoes, or bread is what can make you fat, if you don't choose wisely. Try to stay away from butter, sour cream, and heavy meat sauces.

One of my patients is in the restaurant business, and although she eats plenty of meatless pasta and does not eat butter or desserts, she got into the habit of snacking on prosciutto and cheese, both high in fat and salt. When her weight began to rise, she asked me what to do. Because she was such a sensible eater in general, she was able to lose thirteen pounds in two months just by cutting out the prosciutto and cheese.

Try keeping a written record for two weeks of the foods and fat grams you are eating daily. Note that I want you to do this for only two weeks. Counting fat grams of everything you eat is certainly not how I want you to live. But it helps to have an initial under-standing of how much fat foods contain, and how much, on the average, you are consuming. Once you've attained that sense, the amount of fat in your diet will become second nature.

Keeping such a record is the only way to understand how much fat you are consuming. You will probably be surprised at what you see. If you are a woman consuming approximately 1,800 calories each day, about 360 calories (40 grams) should come from fat. (Each fat gram contains 9 calories.) After a week of record-keeping you should be fully aware of how much fat is in the food you eat. Then you can alter recipes or choose alternative foods to lower the fat content.

I have a patient, a highly educated, accomplished woman in her late forties, who came to me with a triglyceride level of 460. She weighed almost 250 pounds. Here's an idea of her typical daily menu:

Breakfast: two cups of coffee, donuts, and high-sugar cereal
Lunch: Caesar salad with egg and cheese, and dessert
Dinner: High-fat meat and dessert
Late-evening snack: High-fat ice cream

She had a high-pressure job, and the worst high-fat eating binges came during the periods of extreme stress.

She wasn't making much progress when she came to me one day with an announcement: "Dr. Rechtschaffen, I want to lose a lot of weight. I'll do anything you say." (She certainly hadn't before.)

"What's the story?" I asked.

"Dr. Rechtschaffen," she said. "I have a boyfriend!"

Sometimes that's what it takes.

She immediately became conscientious about my recommended diet and activity plan, and she switched to fresh fruit and shredded wheat (or the equivalent) for breakfast. For lunch she had sliced white-meat turkey with lettuce, tomato, and bread, or a vegetable salad with vinaigrette dressing and no-salt crackers. Fish, pasta, or chicken with vegetables became her dinner, and she snacked on fresh fruit instead of ice cream. She also managed to transfer to a less stressful job.

The wedding is planned for June.

Incidentally, another benefit of a low-fat diet—in addition to lowering your risk of heart disease and obesity—is that people who adopt a low-fat diet have fewer feelings of depression and anger.

Eat a Good Breakfast

Breakfast should consist of fresh fruit, complex carbohydrates, and tea or coffee, if you want either. If you're a milk drinker or use milk in your cereal, use skim milk or, at least, low-fat milk.

Actually, low-fat milk is not as low in fat as you would think. Ordinary milk contains about 3 percent fat, so if "low-fat" milk contains 1 or 2 percent fat the difference is almost negligible. Skim milk has taken away most of the fat that's still in low-fat milk. If you insist on using low-fat milk, use 1 percent.

Be as inventive as you can when choosing your breakfast, and don't be limited to typical breakfast foods like packaged cereals. Toast with all-fruit jam or jelly is fine. Some apple-cider jelly made only with apples is also good. When I use all-fruit jam or jelly, I use less than a teaspoonful on a piece of toast. You can also put low-fat cottage cheese on your bread instead of jam.

One of my favorite breakfasts is homemade applesauce with a touch of lemon juice. It's easy to make, and it's a great start to my day, especially with bread and all-fruit jam and a cup of coffee. You can make big batches at a time and store it in the refrigerator.

Many people ask me about eggs. I recommend that you eat no more than two or three eggs a week. Use a nonstick pan and you won't even need butter or anything else to lubricate the pan. Or have boiled or poached eggs. But please don't have cereal, fruit, bread, cheese, all-fruit jam, *and* eggs. Your typical breakfast should be like *one* of the following:

- A whole-grain cereal with skim milk and fruit
- Two slices of bread and an all-fruit spread
- Fresh fruit, egg, and a slice of toast

The possibilities are limitless. (One of my patients likes to microwave pasta with vegetables left over from the previous night's dinner for breakfast, particularly on a cold day.)

We have known for many years that people who eat a good breakfast perform better in school and are more productive at work. Recently, this idea was confirmed by a large study that showed that children who ate breakfast definitely improved their performance in school and increased their IQs. Breakfast eaters also run less risk of overeating later in the day.

One of the reasons that most people have heart attacks in the morning is that they skip breakfast. A recent study shows that tiny particles in the blood called *platelets* stick together in a clump when we don't eat breakfast. We don't know why this happens, but it does. If platelets get out of control, they can cause unwanted and dangerous blood clots. So now you have yet another reason why breakfast is important.

Plan for Healthy Lunches

In order to make sure your lunches are healthy, be sure to pack the following items:

- A vegetable
- A whole grain such as bread, rice, pasta, buckwheat, or couscous (without cream or butter)
- Fish, chicken or turkey breast

And don't forget salads. There's so much you can do with salads and low-fat dressings. If you want to, you can dilute an oil-based dressing with water to cut down on the fat. Remember that lunch should contribute about one quarter of your day's calories.

A sandwich of turkey, lettuce, and tomato on whole-grain bread with mustard is a delicious, healthy lunch. So is a salad of mixed vegetables, or low-fat, low-salt soup and a salad, or soup and half a sandwich, or yogurt and fresh fruit, or low-fat cottage cheese and yogurt mixed with fresh diced vegetables. If you can make and carry your own lunch to work, you can have greater control over what you eat. If you cannot take your own lunch, find restaurants that will serve you food prepared the way you request it.

55

Eat More Bread

Whole-grain bread is good for you, as long as you don't eat it with butter or other high-fat spreads, or use it to make salami sandwiches. Bread eaten in moderation (two to four slices a day) is not fattening, and it can help you feel satisfied without adding too many calories.

In case you're confused about the difference between whole-wheat bread and other kinds, I'll try to clarify it. On top of each stalk of wheat are several flowerlike clusters. Each cluster is a *kernel*, or one *whole grain*. A whole grain contains the following parts: (1) *fiber-rich bran*; (2) *the germ*, which provides vitamins, minerals, and protein; and (3) the *endosperm*, which is mostly starch. White bread is made from kernels that have had the bran and germ removed, leaving only the starchy endosperm. As a result, white bread has little nutritional value.

Incidentally, some perfectly good meals may leave you feeling hungry if you don't also have a slice or two of bread. For example, one of my patients recently prepared a very nice dinner of chicken breasts, brussels sprouts, and an apple-celeriac-walnut salad. The entire family loved the meal, but they were still hungry afterward. A slice or two of whole-grain bread with the salad would have solved the problem.

56

Make Brown Bagging and Take-outs Work for You

More than half of the working adults in the United States "brown bag" it regularly. I hope to give you a few ideas to pack a nutritious meal when you carry your lunch to work, or when you order take-out food and eat it at your desk.

For a small investment of your time in the morning (or the night before), you can have a great homemade lunch *and* save money. And I promise you will be more alert and productive after a good, healthy lunch instead of a hot dog and soda. One of the real advantages of taking your own lunch is being able to have hot or cold homemade soup. Wide-mouthed thermos bottles have been designed to carry soup and other semiliquid foods such as chili or stew. I have a Chinese friend who takes homemade Chinese food to work and eats it at his desk, in the company cafeteria, or in the local park. Cold soup, including gazpacho, is a real treat on a hot day (see the recipe on page 205).

If you want a chicken or turkey (without skin, preferably white-meat) sandwich on whole-grain bread with lettuce and tomato, pack the lettuce and tomato separately from the sandwich so the bread won't get soggy. Pasta salad is another good choice. It is nutritious as well as satisfying, and it travels well. Also try potato salad with a low-fat vinaigrette dressing or a yogurt dressing that you add later. (See the recipes for these dressings on pages 214 and 215.)

Low-fat, low-salt cheese is excellent for brown bagging. Nibble on some fresh raw vegetables with the cheese, and add a few low-fat, low-salt whole-grain crackers and fresh juice, mineral water, tea, or coffee. Use skim or low-fat milk if you ordinarily drink your tea or coffee with milk. Water-packed tuna is always a good idea, either eaten plain or as part of a vinaigrette vegetable salad.

By all means, don't forget to pack fresh fruit and a plain bagel or whole-grain bread. Another idea is low-fat, low-salt dips with fresh carrots, celery, broccoli, and cauliflower. If you need to keep your lunch cold, you can buy an insulated lunch tote, pack a cold can of juice to provide extra coolness, or use special nondrip ice packs that you store in your home freezer.

When you are ordering a take-out meal, try to avoid cold cuts or the usual hamburger, french fries, and soda. The majority of restaurants are now geared to prepare and deliver take-out orders, and you have a greater variety of food to choose from than ever before. You don't even have to settle for a sandwich anymore. French, Greek, Italian, Oriental, and other types of food are also awaiting your phone call or fax. Make sure to tell the restaurant to avoid fatty dressings, monosodium glutamate (MSG), salt, soy sauce, and all the other things you wouldn't order in a restaurant. You will be surprised at how accommodating most restaurants can be. Just tell them what you're trying to accomplish, and they'll usually prepare a so-called light meal to your specifications.

The same is true of airlines. You do not have to eat whatever is served on an airplane. Make arrangements ahead for a healthy meal, including vegetarian fare and other special requests. Or bring your own light snack—I always do. Airline passengers are generally envious of someone who has brought good, *fresh* food on a flight. (I'm not talking about bringing a chicken dinner!)

57

Keep the Fruits and Their Juices

The current "juicing mania" does not take into account an important dietary element of fresh fruits and vegetables: their natural fiber. Juices are very good, but the fruits and vegetables you squeeze and throw away may be even better, because they contain lots of fiber, which you should be eating. Also, watch the calories in fruit juices. The count may be higher than you think. Instead of drinking the juice of three or four pieces of fruit, eat one piece of fruit instead.

If you are squeezing your own fruit or vegetable juice (and I hope you are), use a juicer that retains as much of the pulp as possible.

58

Get More Carotene and Vitamin C

V itamins A and C both seem to help prevent some cancers. Dark green, leafy vegetables such as spinach and broccoli, yellow vegetables such as squash and carrots, and fruits contain relatively large amounts of carotene, a chemical the body converts into vitamin A. Excellent sources of vitamin C are citrus fruits, green peppers, sweet red peppers, tomatoes, and potatoes.

Eat more of these foods:

Food	Carotene	Vitamin C
Apricots	High	Medium
Broccoli	High	High
Brussels sprouts	Medium	High
Cantaloupe	High	High
Carrots	High	Medium
Citrus fruits	Low	High
Dark green, leafy vegetables	High	Medium
Green peppers	Medium	High
Peaches	High	Medium
Peas	Medium	High
Squash	High	Medium
Strawberries	Low	High
Sweet potatoes	High	High
Tomatoes	High	High

I recommend a daily vitamin C supplement of 2 to 3 grams (2,000 to 3,000 milligrams). If you don't mind the extra expense, buy calcium ascorbate as a source of vitamin C, because the calcium acts as a buffer that reduces gastrointestinal irritation, and the extra calcium may help relieve osteoporosis (a decrease in bone mass and density). If calcium ascorbate is too expensive, use ascorbic acid, but not sodium ascorbate, which contains more sodium than you need.

I do not recommend taking a vitamin A supplement, because unlike vitamin C, vitamin A builds up in the body instead of being eliminated in the urine if not needed. Excessive amounts of vitamin A can have dangerous side effects. Also, diabetics should consult their physicians before increasing their intake of vitamin A or carotene-rich food. (See "Vitamins and Minerals: Are You Getting Enough?" on page 180.)

59

Eat Well to Help Prevent Skin Cancer

Here's a little-known connection between cancer and a low-fat diet: Skin cancer is by far the most common type of cancer, with about a million cases diagnosed in the United States each year. The incidence of sunlight-caused skin cancer and its common forerunner—a lesion called *actinic keratosis*—may be reduced by as much as 60 percent if you eat a low-fat diet.

60

Check for Your Own Fiber Deficiency

When someone is not receiving enough protein, we say that he or she has a protein deficiency. But when a person is not getting enough fiber, we don't think of it as a deficiency. We should. According to the National Cancer Institute, we need 20 to 35 grams of fiber a day.

Too many people in the United States are suffering from a deficiency of fiber that could be corrected rather easily. Next to water, unprocessed bran is probably your best bargain. A half-pound of packaged unprocessed bran costs less than two dollars and lasts a month; 100 caplets of 1,000-milligram oat bran costs less than five dollars and lasts longer than a month.

Besides helping you avoid many gastrointestinal problems, three to four tablespoons (two to three caplets) of bran each day will help you lose weight by filling you without adding significant calories. (Each caplet of oat bran contains 4 calories.) Make sure you drink six to eight glasses of water every day to assist the action of the bran in giving you proper bowel movements. You may find that you get a little "gassy" on a high-fiber diet, but that will settle down after two or three weeks.

A half cup of cooked brussels sprouts contains about 5 grams of fiber, making sprouts one of the highest-fiber vegetables. The calorie count is only about 30, yet you still get significant amounts of vitamins C, A, and B.

Eat more of these foods:

1. *Whole-grain foods,* including Wheatena, farina, whole-grain oatmeal, pure shredded wheat, rice, pasta, grits, buckwheat or kasha, and couscous
2. *Whole-grain breads,* including whole-wheat; oatmeal; wheat-germ; unsalted whole-wheat Melba toast; pita bread; whole-wheat bran matzoh
3. *Raw fruit,* with skin
4. *Leafy and raw vegetables,* with skin
5. *Unprocessed bran* (wheat, rice, or oat), preferably three to four tablespoons a day, not necessarily all at once. Bran is also available in a convenient pill form. Drink plenty of water with bran
6. *Water,* at least six to eight glasses a day

The Center for Science in the Public Interest recently ranked the top ten fruits on the basis of nutrient and fiber content. The fruits are, from the top: papaya, cantaloupe, strawberry, orange, tangerine, kiwi, mango, apricot, persimmon, and watermelon.

61

Help Keep Your
Digestive Tract Healthy

Eating a variety of fiber-rich foods, including whole-grain breads and cereals, fresh fruits and vegetables, beans, and nuts, helps prevent constipation and other gastrointestinal disorders such as diverticulosis. Constipation is virtually nonexistent with a high-fiber diet, which may also prevent diarrhea. In other words, a high-fiber diet does not disrupt your body—just the opposite. It allows your body to function as a well-balanced mechanism, the way it is meant to. A high-fiber, low-fat diet may help lower cholesterol, control blood sugar in diabetics, and prevent colon, prostate, and breast cancer.

One of my most dramatic cases involving a high-fiber diet involved a forty-four-year-old man who had suffered with diarrhea since he was thirteen. He followed the high-fiber diet I prescribed, and he has been having normal, healthy, regular bowel movements ever since. Another case comes to mind because my patient had exactly the opposite problem: he had had chronic constipation and bloating for over a year. He was a fast-food junkie who loved diet sodas and always looked forward to having a pastry at coffee breaks. He began eating a low-fat, low-sugar, high-complex-carbohydrate, high-fiber diet, with some extra apple bran for a couple of weeks, and now he has regular bowel movements and has given up his junk-food mania. Because the constipation, gas, and bloating are gone for good, he feels better and looks forward to his sensible meals and snacks.

If you are over fifty years old, your chances of getting hemorrhoids are about fifty-fifty. When you are constipated, you inadvertently cause side effects such as hemorrhoids by straining during defecation. You put too much pressure on your rectum and large intestine, and cause their small blood vessels to balloon. When you begin to take the daily three to four tablespoons of unprocessed bran or bran caplets that I recommend, you will probably do away with constipation, diarrhea, hemorrhoids, and anal itching at the same time. It sounds impossible, doesn't it? But it's true.

By the way, since we're talking about bloating, let me give you a couple of tips to help avoid that painful and embarrassing problem. First, visit your physician to find out whether you have a lactose intolerance, which can cause severe bloating and pain. The same symptoms may be caused by sulfites in wine and wine sauces. Drink plenty of water with your bran to ease constipation and bloating, and do not sit in the same position for long periods of time right after dinner. One of the reasons a postdinner walk is such a good idea is that it gives your food a chance to move downward along your digestive tract without getting scrunched up, as when you are sitting. One of my patients would always arrive home in pain after visiting a relative two and a half hours away by car. The routine was always the same: He would go out to dinner with his relative and then get into his car and drive home immediately afterward. By the time he got home, his abdominal area was so swollen that he had to undo his belt buckle and open his pants, and he could barely walk from his car to his house.

If you respect your body and understand the essentials of how it works, it will perform at its maximum potential, with the least amount of trouble.

62

Reduce Your Salt Intake

If your physician can control the amount of salt in your diet, he or she can probably control your blood pressure. More than that, he or she can probably lower your blood pressure if it is too high. Usually, atherosclerosis and high blood pressure are both *reversible through diet.*

One of my patients is Craig Claiborne, the eminent food writer. I first met him about fifteen years ago when he came to me with very high blood pressure. One of my first questions was, "Do you eat a lot of salt?" His answer was, "Salt? I'm addicted to the stuff."

It turns out that Mr. Claiborne had been eating salty, fatty foods since his southern childhood. I put him on a low-salt, low-fat, low-sugar, high-fiber, high-complex-carbohydrate diet, and within three months he had lost almost thirty pounds. His blood pressure dropped from 186/112 to 140/80, a normal range. Mr. Claiborne also began walking instead of taking taxis, and he was feeling better than ever. Here's what he has to say about the program he adopted: "To achieve my present good health it was not necessary to alter my lifestyle dramatically, so much as to acquaint myself with a proper program of physical activity and diet—a diet I enjoy without a feeling of deprivation."

About twenty-five million Americans suffer from high blood pressure. It is sometimes called "the silent disease" because it usually is already a problem before any indication shows up. Before you know it, a heart attack or cerebral hemorrhage can strike. The only real way to detect high blood pressure early is to have regular checkups that include your blood pressure. By the way, it is a myth that your blood pressure is normal if it equals your age plus 100. In most cases such a number would be too high.

Why does salt intake increase blood pressure? Salt in your blood attracts and retains fluid. This increases the amount of blood in your blood vessels at any given time. Salt also causes hormonal changes that may reduce the size of the opening of the arteries. If the same amount of blood is to be pumped to all parts of your body, the pressure must be increased to keep the blood moving through the smaller opening. (It's the same phenomenon that causes the water to spray out of a garden hose in a firmer, more distant stream when you partially block the nozzle with your finger. The smaller the opening, the greater the fluid pressure.)

If you eat a lot of salt, you probably find that you feel thirsty. It's not just the salty taste in your mouth that's making you feel thirsty. Your body is telling you to drink more liquid in an effort to dilute the salt so you can finally eliminate it in your urine.

Almost 80 percent of the sodium in most people's diets comes from processed foods. With this in mind, there are two things you can do: (1) Cut down on the salt you add to food so you can counteract the huge amount already in processed foods, and (2) Use fewer processed foods and read the labels more carefully when you do use them. In addition to watching out for sodium, be wary of foods that contain hidden sodium, such as baking powder, baking soda, monosodium glutamate, sodium benzoate, and other ingredients with *sodium* in their names.

In cultures where no salt is used, people do not have high blood pressure, and blood pressure does not increase with age, as it does in this country. In contrast, American children of parents who die of cardiovascular disease before the age of fifty are likely to show early signs of their own cardiovascular problems. The chances of high blood fat in these young children can be as high as 50 percent. The normal possibility is one half of one percent—*100 times less.*

But even if you don't inherit a tendency toward cardiovascular disease, you may still be setting up problems early in your life. Children who eat snacks containing large amounts of sugar and salt may be conditioned for future cases of high blood pressure and other forms of cardiovascular disease. People who consume large amounts of salt and sugar have also been known to suffer more from osteoporosis and generally weakened bones than those who do not. This situation is aggravated by too little physical activity—a harmful trend among today's children. It's bad enough that children are snacking on high-salt, high-calorie junk food, but they are doing it while *sitting* for hours in front of television sets.

Change the trend—if not for your sake, then for the sake of your children.

63 ◆ Have Regular Checkups

Recently I found two cases of lung cancer through ordinary chest X rays during annual physical exams. You can prevent many serious problems from developing if you catch them early, during regular annual checkups. Regular breast examinations for women are a must, as are regular prostate checkups for men, including a PSA (prostate-specific antigen) blood test. You'd be amazed at what your physician can detect during a complete physical examination.

I have a patient who developed pneumonia. In the normal course of checking his blood, I found high levels of triglycerides, cholesterol, and sugar. If he had had regular checkups, these problems would have been found and treated sooner. Incidentally, this was a young man who used to carry candy in his pockets and snack all day long. He doesn't do that anymore.

64

Stop Smoking

Cigarette smoking is just plain bad for you. The surgeon general's reminder on each pack of cigarettes should be enough to get you to stop smoking. (Would you continue to eat a food that contained all those warnings?) There is *no doubt* that smoking causes lung cancer; may cause birth defects; aggravates atherosclerosis, arthritis, and lung conditions such as asthma; and harms your body in many other ways. And besides the life-threatening aspects of smoking, it also makes your skin wrinkled, your taste buds inefficient, and your breath unpleasant. (Clark Gable's leadings ladies hated to work with him because his cigarette breath smelled so bad.)

Smoking is also unfair to the people around you, especially children. There is hard evidence that "second-hand smoke" kills about three thousand people a year.

Incidentally, if you are a smoker, you can decrease your chances of having emphysema and chronic pulmonary disease by eating fish a few times a week.

But better yet, stop smoking.

65

Be Flexible
during Holidays

If you normally eat a low-fat diet, you don't have to worry about what to eat on Thanksgiving and other holidays. Relax, and enjoy the pumpkin pie.

But I will caution you that if you have been following a low-fat diet and then you overindulge on Thanksgiving with lots of fatty foods, you could be in for some serious gastrointestinal distress. Why? Because you will be throwing your system out of balance by suddenly eating a high-fat meal.

If you do want to cut some fat out of your holiday dinner, try a bulgur or rice and vegetable stuffing (see the recipe on page 210), and ignore the turkey skin and dark meat. Skip the candied sweet potatoes and creamed onions altogether, and enjoy a moderate portion of dessert. Try vegetables prepared with herbs and lemon juice. Be creative. There are many low-fat ways to prepare holiday foods that are just as tasty (tastier to me) and festive as the higher-fat versions. For example, I personally don't think marshmallows add anything to sweet potatoes.

Here is another low-fat tip: Baste the turkey with low-fat, low-salt broth or stock. (To reduce the fat in broth: Chill broth in your refrigerator overnight, and then remove it and discard the solidified fat at the top.) In my family, we always make our own fresh cranberry relish sweetened with a little orange juice, cinnamon sticks, and cloves.

Do not make an issue over what you can or cannot eat. Enjoy the holidays and just try not to *over*-overeat. To compensate, take longer walks than usual for the rest of the week.

Choose the Best
Times to Exercise

When is the best time to exercise? Whenever you can. But exercise *before* meals burns the most body fat because your glycogen stores are low, and your body tends to burn fat to conserve glycogen. (Glycogen is the stored form of glucose.) The combination of walking before meals and eating a low-fat, high-complex-carbohydrate diet leads to the quickest and greatest weight loss. A low-fat, high-complex-carbohydrate diet replaces glycogen without replacing fat.

Because your glycogen storage is at its lowest before breakfast, any physical activity before breakfast leads to the greatest burning of body fat. There is no better way to get your day off to a good start than with a long walk. It warms your body, limbers up your muscles, feeds your senses, and jump-starts your brain.

Eat Well When
You're on the Run

Only about 20 percent of us eat three meals a day. The remaining 80 percent usually skip breakfast or lunch, snack a lot, and are barely interested in the nutritive value of food. Unfortunately, it's typical of busy people to eat on the run. Indeed, we may very well be the only land animals that willingly move and eat at the same time.

I would prefer that you eat your meals quietly and peacefully, but if you are on the go most of the time and *really* can't change that pattern, I would rather change *what* you eat than *how* you eat.

A person on the run in a big city might typically eat the following lunch on the way from one appointment to another: Frankfurter (with mustard and sauerkraut), a twelve-ounce can of soda, and a candy bar. The chances are good that two blocks later there will be another frankfurter vendor, and we can add another hot dog to the menu. Total calories: 710.

Assuming the usual availability of storefront merchants and street vendors, here is a meal-on-the-run that I would recommend instead: One slice of pizza (preferably vegetable pizza, without cheese), one cup of freshly squeezed orange juice or eight ounces of mineral water (without sodium), one apple (or whatever fresh fruit is available), and a handful of dry-roasted, unsalted almonds. Total calories: 470.

Let's take a closer look at the two meals. The lunch of frank-furters, soda, and candy was high in sugar, fat, and salt, and low in complex carbohydrates and fiber. It had little or no nutritional value, and it stimulated the appetite. Instead of providing energy, the high sugar content of the meal actually produced fatigue.

The second meal was not perfect either, but it certainly was better. It provided real energy in the form of complex carbohydrates, and it was high in fiber. Unlike the first meal, it did not stimulate the appetite; it was also lower in calories, and it contained relatively low amounts of simple sugar, fat, and salt.

By the way, even if you are in a hurry, you don't have to gulp down your food. Eat as slowly as you can, and try to relax and enjoy it. Always *eat slowly*. The faster you eat, the more you will eat, and the sooner you will be hungry again.

Here are some alternatives to a typical high-sugar meal-on-the-run:

Try to Avoid	Have Instead
Hot dogs	Pizza (1 slice; preferably vegetable pizza, without cheese)
Hamburgers	Falafel
	Shishkebab
	Plain hamburger (with lettuce and tomato, if desired)
Soda	Freshly squeezed orange juice
	Mineral water
	Seltzer (which is low-salt)
Candy	Fresh fruit
Ice cream	No-fat, no-sugar frozen yogurt
	No-fat, no-sugar yogurt drink

Try to Avoid	*Have Instead*
Salted pretzel	Toasted plain bagel
	Breadsticks (low-salt, low-fat)
	Matzoh (low-salt)
Peanuts	Air-popped, unbuttered, unsalted popcorn (the calories in one cup of peanuts—840—are equal to the calories in thirty-two cups of plain popcorn)

Fight the Fatness Moguls

Every year the food industry in the United States spends about $36 *billion* on ads meant to get you to eat more of its products than you need. Much of that advertising appears on television. In my opinion, watching television—coupled with snacking—is one of the worst culprits in the fight against obesity and poor health. Most adults watch between four and five hours of television a day, a lot of it right after dinner—not a good time to be sedentary.

In 1994, Dr. Michael Jacobson, the executive director of the Center for Science in the Public Interest, suggested that the Clinton administration sponsor an annual national "No-TV Week," which would encourage physical activity instead of television watching. Not a bad idea.

A friend of mine from France visited me here recently, and he made a telling remark that I would like to share with you. "No wonder Americans are so fat," he said. "They are eating all the time."

Obesity is not as big a problem in France as it is here, for several reasons that I can see. For one, French people usually do not snack between meals. Also, they eat smaller portions than we do, and they frequently make lunch their main meal. It also seems to me that they walk more than we do and are more physically active in general.

I was watching the World Cup soccer matches on television recently, and I noticed that there were no intermissions except during halftime. This means that the typical French viewer is not going to make a trip to the kitchen every ten minutes or so, the way many Americans do who watch baseball, football, or basketball games, with their innumerable delays and sponsor-controlled "television time-outs."

All in all, we eat too much and sit too much. We are letting the food advertisers win the battle, and we aren't even putting up a decent fight.

Get Rid of That Tired Feeling

Many people claim they are tired all the time. They go to bed tired, and they wake up tired. Obviously, something is wrong, and they should check with their physicians to make sure they don't have a physical or emotional problem, such as chronic fatigue syndrome or depression. Here are some things that might be making you tired without you being aware of them:

1. You may be bored. Is your work stimulating? Is *anything* stimulating? When was the last time you took a satisfying, restful, rejuvenating vacation?

2. When you are tired in the afternoon and you think you need a snack to pick you up, don't eat or drink anything that contains caffeine or sugar, including coffee, soda, candy, or cookies. Although such foods may make you feel better for a short time, the overall effect will be greater fatigue. Try complex carbohydrates instead, such as a plain bagel, fresh vegetables, a few low-salt, low-fat crackers, or a piece of fresh fruit. (The sugar in a piece of fruit is not as concentrated as it is in a glass of juice because the fruit contains pulp and other solids.)

3. Many people are completely sedentary. *They* say they are sedentary because they are tired. *I* say they are tired because they are not allowing their bodies to be active. A daily walk at a brisk

pace will help you feel awake and alive—and you'll sleep better and eat less too.

4. Drink six to eight glasses of water every day. Water will help to keep you from getting drowsy, will prevent the debilitating effects of dehydration, and will keep you healthy in many other ways. The next time you think you are hungry between meals, drink a glass of cool water instead of eating food. It will satisfy you without adding pounds.

5. Sleep with the heat off and the windows open, and make sure you are not working in an overheated room. A little ventilation will perk you up.

6. Get interested in something that you can look forward to doing every day. I know that may not be easy, but it's very important.

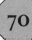

Add Flavor
without Adding Salt

Many of my patients frown when I tell them to lower their intake of salt. My food will be so *boring,* they say. Not so. Here are a few ways to spice up your food either by using considerably less salt or by not using salt in any form.

Try using a home-cooked, unsalted tomato sauce (see the recipe on page 207) to add taste to such foods as veal, chicken, pasta, or rice. Become acquainted with scallions, shallots, leeks, garlic, onions, and chives to enliven salads, sauces, soups, yogurt, meat, and fish. Fresh horseradish is delicious with cold salads, fish, and many other foods. You can find fresh horseradish in most fruit markets.

Enjoy fresh fruit for meals and for between-meal treats. Bits of fresh fruit can be an appealing taste enhancer when added to yogurt, cereal, salads, and other foods.

The flavor of cooked food can be accentuated with a sprinkling of herbs such as rosemary, garlic, tarragon, basil, or parsley. You might also try oregano, marjoram, mustard (salt-free, if possible), tumeric, chervil, whole peppers, or a combination of basil, parsley, and oregano. Try a dash of paprika for a nice touch of color.

Pepper in its many forms, vinegar, and lemon or lime juice are other flavorful additions to a meal. Top off salads, oatmeal, rice, yogurt, cottage cheese, corn and other fresh vegetables with freshly ground pepper, but *not salt.* Use vinegar and peppercorns on sautéed fish or veal. Squeeze lemon juice and sprinkle pepper on cauliflower or broccoli. Try crushed red pepper on eggplant spread, pasta, cauliflower, pureed vegetables such as broccoli and cauliflower, and on grated zucchini. Sprinkle a dab of cayenne powder on top of fish, veal, chicken, and casseroles or stews. (Cayenne pepper is very hot and should be used sparingly.) Incidentally, red and green peppers are excellent sources of vitamin C.

A mixture of vinegar and dill makes a great topping for tomatoes and other fresh vegetables. A dressing of lemon juice, vinegar, and dill or tarragon or rosemary adds zest to plain broiled meat and fish or salads, and to fresh vegetables such as green beans, brussels sprouts, tomatoes, and potatoes. Vinegar or lemon juice is a superb addition to almost any fresh vegetable. When sprinkled on a food, each one adds zest to the flavor so that you need far less salt, if any.

If you use your imagination, you won't need much salt.

Think about
Salad Dressings

You can ruin a healthy salad by dousing it with a fatty dressing. Make your own dressing. Try this:

    3 tablespoons of olive oil
    1 tablespoon of vinegar
    1 teaspoon of prepared mustard
    a pinch of dried parsley, oregano, and basil
    3 tablespoons of water

Two tablespoons of this dressing provide only 6 grams of fat because you have diluted the oil.

This vinaigrette dressing can be used in a hundred ways—as salad dressing, a marinade or basting liquid for baked or broiled fish or chicken, a light sauce for steamed vegetables, or a topping for a baked potato.

◇ 72 ◇

Cook Ahead

Everything is more enjoyable when you have the time to do it well. Dinnertime is often a family's most frenetic time, with people coming from school or work and getting ready for social activities. Sometimes it's hard to concentrate on *anything*, much less cooking and eating well. So if cooking has become another time-consuming job wedged into an already hectic workday, the tendency for "quick fixes" or fast food might prove tempting.

One way around that is to plan a week's worth of menus over the weekend (with your partner, if you have one). With main courses made and frozen, each night's dinner preparation can be reduced to making a salad or cooking fresh vegetables. Cooking can then become almost a leisure activity, one that can be done together on weekends, when you have time, rather than each night, when time is short and you are tired.

One of my patients works long hours and doesn't have time to cook in the evenings, but she enjoys cooking large batches of food on the weekend and using them all week long. The only problem was, she cooked fried chicken, bacon, fatty pork, and other salty and fatty foods. When I persuaded her to change that pattern, her weight dropped from 193 to 147 in eight months, and she has maintained a healthy weight, along with a new, healthy lifestyle. And she still cooks on weekends for weekday meals.

Let Restaurants Know
What You Want

There's an old expression that says, "If you can open your mouth to eat, you can also open it to speak." Don't be intimidated in a restaurant; ask questions and make special requests. For example, if the menu offers broiled filet of sole with a cream sauce, ask the waiter to leave off the sauce and bring lots of fresh lemon instead.

I have found that it's important *how* you ask for changes in the menu. If you are polite and are genuinely interested in food, the waiter will be happy to help you. But if you demand changes in a critical way, you can expect little cooperation.

In certain cases it's best to stick with the selections on the menu. A good rule to follow is this: Do not go to a four-star, internationally acclaimed restaurant and ask them to make major adjustments for you. That would be like buying a $3,000 dress and then having it redesigned. Let's face it, you don't go to a four-star restaurant every day. So when you do go, make the most sensible choices, but also make sure you have a great time. That doesn't mean you have to order every rich food on the menu, but it does mean you can have the filet of sole *with* the cream sauce if that's the specialty of the house.

When you're dining out with friends, one way to avoid the problem of an overflowing plate is to share several appetizers instead of having a typical main course. Seek out restaurants that offer an interesting variety of appetizers. Not only will you be eating less than if you ordered one appetizer and a main course just for yourself, but the sharing itself is a wonderful way to make the event a social success. I have not had any difficulty with sharing appetizers in a restaurant. In fact, waiters seem pleased to accommodate the suggestion.

Cook with Wine

One way to cut down on fat and salt—and to increase the flavor of your food without adding calories—is to cook with a combination of wine, herbs, and succulent vegetables to create a flavor that goes beyond the capabilities of salt. But doesn't cooking with wine add all the calories of the alcohol? The answer is no. An especially welcome feature of cooking with wine is that most of the alcohol and calories in the wine burn off during cooking, but the enriching flavor of the wine remains.

When you cook, you do not need to use an expensive wine—in fact, it would be wasteful. At the same time, inferior wines contribute only poor taste to your food, so use an inexpensive but reliable table wine from a reputable vintner and shipper. (Learn to read a wine label, if you don't know how to already.) And by all means, *do not* use "cooking wines"—they contain lots of salt.

75

Avoid Pickled
and Smoked Foods

Salt-cured and smoked foods have been implicated in cancer of the stomach and esophagus (the tube leading from the mouth to the stomach). Avoid foods that contain nitrite and nitrate preservatives, because those chemicals are converted into carcinogenic, or cancer-causing, nitrosamines. Foods that contain hydrocarbons, which are thought to be carcinogenic, should also be avoided.

Specifically, avoid these foods:

Bacon
Bologna
Frankfurters
Ham
Sausages
Smoked fish

Eat Plenty of Garlic

Garlic and onions have been used as home remedies for thousands of years, but now there is scientific evidence that they may actually act as "antibiotics" and help prevent cancer and cardiovascular disease. Apparently, the sulfur compounds in garlic and onions contain the disease-fighting components.

Use fresh garlic cloves when you cook—no dried garlic powder, and no garlic press either. (A garlic press squeezes out most of the juice and much of the flavor.) Smash a clove on your work surface with the side of a heavy knife, lift away the peel, then chop up the garlic, and presto—minced garlic. Too-high heat destroys the true flavor of garlic, making it bitter. So never put garlic under the broiler or sauté it in oil that's too hot. Generally it is best to add garlic to the liquid in a sauce, stew, or soup just a few minutes before the dish is to be served.

Put a Sweet Red Pepper in Your Salad

What are the best sources of vitamin C? Citrus fruits? Here's a surprise: 1 medium raw sweet red pepper contains as much vitamin C as 1 medium orange, and 3$^1/_2$ times the vitamin C in half a grapefruit. In descending order, here are some excellent sources of vitamin C in normal servings:

Raw sweet red pepper (1 medium)
Cantaloupe ($^1/_2$)
Broccoli (1 cup, cooked)
Brussels sprouts (1 cup, cooked)
Raw green pepper (1 medium)
Papaya ($^1/_2$)
Strawberries (1 cup)
Kiwifruit (1 medium)
Orange (1 medium)
Grapefruit ($^1/_2$)

And sweet peppers taste so good!

Learn How a Healthy Lifestyle Helps Prevent Diabetes

The effect of nutrition and physical activity on our lives is enormous. We can and must take charge of our bodies to increase our chances of having a healthy, long life. Maintaining a healthy weight is a critical part of a natural disease-prevention program.

One of the diseases that can be prevented is adult-onset diabetes (a form of diabetes that affects only adults), which is not necessarily related to an insulin deficiency and is usually less severe than juvenile-onset diabetes. Eating a low-fat, high-complex-carbohydrate diet, coupled with a moderate aerobic exercise program performed on a regular basis, is the best way to prevent adult-onset diabetes. Elderly adults who do twenty minutes of physical activity three times a week may reduce the incidence or severity of type II adult-onset diabetes.

Women with diabetes have three to four times the risk of developing heart disease or suffering a stroke as do women without diabetes. Although we know that the tendency to contract diabetes may be hereditary, we do not know why women with diabetes are more susceptible to heart disease and strokes.

79

Start Your Day with the Right "Instant" Breakfast

Now that the dual-income family has become the norm in American life, there is even less time for cooking than before. Breakfast seems to be the meal that suffers most, since lunch is eaten out and a quick dinner can always be prepared or ordered out for the family.

Breakfast is an important meal, and I wish everyone had the time and inclination to have a good breakfast every day. But many people don't like to eat in the morning (these same people are famished by the time the coffee cart comes around, so they eat pastries and whatever else is available), or they just don't have time to prepare anything. Incidentally, about 12 percent of all sodas are consumed in the *morning*. I have a few suggestions that may improve on soda for breakfast.

Here are some simple recipes for nutritious and delicious breakfast drinks that will send you out of the house feeling contented rather than hungry. If you can, also have a piece of toast, a plain half bagel, or half a matzoh with your drink. Also, use these drinks as "pep-up" drinks instead of snacking in the afternoon, and by all means experiment with your own combinations of fruits and juices. Vanilla protein powder can be obtained in any health-food store; make sure it's a low-fat, low-sugar, low-salt type.

BANANA-STRAWBERRY BREAKFAST DRINK

$^1/_2$ banana, sliced
3 to 4 frozen whole strawberries
1 heaping teaspoon vanilla protein powder, without added sugar
1 teaspoon vanilla extract
$^1/_2$ cup cold skim or low-fat milk

Place ingredients in a blender and run on Liquefy setting for about a minute, until the mixture is smooth and creamy. Pour into a clear glass and drink immediately, while it is still cold and fresh.

SUMMERTIME BREAKFAST DRINK

$^1/_4$ cup fresh or frozen blueberries
$^1/_4$ banana, sliced
1 fresh peach or nectarine, cubed
3 fresh or frozen strawberries
1 heaping teaspoon vanilla protein powder, without added sugar
1 teaspoon vanilla extract
$^1/_4$ cup cold skim or low-fat milk

Place ingredients in a blender and run on Liquefy setting for about a minute, or until the mixture is smooth and creamy. Pour into a clear glass and drink immediately, while it is still cold and fresh.

ORANGE-STRAWBERRY FRAPPÉ

6 frozen sections of fresh navel orange; peel, section, and freeze
   an orange the night before
3 frozen whole strawberries
$1/4$ cup fresh orange juice
$1/4$ cup cold skim or low-fat milk
2 ice cubes

Blend to a creamy froth in blender. Top with a sprig of parsley if you want to add an attractive touch.

APPLE-BANANA SMOOTHIE

1 small to medium apple, unpeeled, quartered
$1/2$ banana, sliced
$1/4$ cup apple juice, no sugar added
$1/4$ cup cold skim or low-fat milk
2 ice cubes

Blend until smooth in blender. Sprinkle with nutmeg.

80

Follow a Healthy Diet during Pregnancy

I tell all my pregnant patients that they are absolutely correct to think they should be eating for two during their pregnancy. But—and this is an important but—remember that the second person is small and brand new, without any bad habits to break. This is a parent's chance to start that baby off with the best possible gift of positive living even before birth.

When you are pregnant, it is normal to think about your every action in terms of how it will affect your baby. Take the time now to reflect on the health, comfort, development, and nutritional, psychological, and physical needs of your unborn child. Offer your child a wide selection of the best natural foods—plenty of fresh vegetables and fruits, whole grains, and high-quality protein. You and the baby need more protein now than at any other time of your lives.

What an opportunity: a clean slate. Don't mar it. Take good care of that baby, starting now. Don't smoke, don't drink alcohol, get plenty of rest and low-impact exercise, and eat only the best nutritional foods. When you do, you will be giving your child the healthiest chance at a good life, and you will feel so much healthier yourself that you will most likely maintain a healthy, nutritional lifestyle after the baby is born.

Eat Plenty of Pasta

Pasta—whether dried or fresh—has no fat, is low in calories (210 per five ounces cooked), is an excellent source of complex carbohydrates, and is enriched with vitamins and iron. The best dried pasta is made from durum wheat (semolina) combined with a small amount of flour. That wonderful firm texture of properly cooked pasta comes from the semolina.

Pasta alone contains no fat. As I've been saying, the fat comes from the sauces or cheese you put on it. Try a plain tomato sauce or pureed fresh vegetables with pasta, or use grilled fresh vegetables with a little chicken for a delicious, nutritious low-fat high-complex-carbohydrate meal. (See pages 207 and 208 for some recipes.)

And remember, you can increase the portion of pasta itself without additional sauce and not consume additional fat. If you had pasta with a tomato sauce or with fresh vegetables two or three times a week, you would be well on the road to healthy eating.

Treat Yourself to a Nap

More and more research tells us that a midday nap is a good idea. If you are at home, take a thirty-minute break and lie down, without feeling guilty. (Don't watch television or do anything else during this time; just relax.) If you're at the office and can't lie down or put your head down at your desk, relax in a restroom cubicle or a designated rest area for ten or fifteen minutes. Even a short period of total relaxation will make you feel more efficient when you return to your chores. It will also keep you from falling asleep soon after lunch; an after-lunch nap or a nap too late in the afternoon may make it difficult to sleep at bedtime.

Too many of us are running around so much that we give up sleep in order to do other things. Each person needs a different amount of sleep, and you should respect your own needs, but make sure you get enough sleep. Sleep loss can reduce the number of some disease-fighting immune cells in your immune system. On the other hand, some of us are getting *too much* sleep. Don't fall into the trap of staying in bed very late every morning—it isn't healthy (it will cause you to eat irregularly, and will slow down your metabolism), and it may indicate that you are using sleep to hide from something you don't want to face.

Incidentally, drinking alcohol or eating late at night will not help you sleep—just the opposite.

Be Picky about Packaged Cereals

Children don't choose a breakfast cereal because of its nutritional value; they choose it because of a television commercial that contains an interesting cartoon character or a catchy jingle. Most of those cereals are loaded with sugar. Here are some examples: Quaker 100% Natural Oats & Honey contains seven teaspoons of sugar per cup of cereal. (Here's a good case of deceptive advertising that can really hurt you. Many of us have been conditioned to think of the words *natural, oats,* and *honey* as good. The word *natural* usually doesn't mean much and provides an opportunity for the manufacturer to use so-called natural sugar; oats are okay, as long as you don't cover them with sugar; and honey is just another form of sugar.)

Here is the sugar content of some other popular cereals:

Cereal	*Teaspoons of Sugar per Cup of Cereal*
Kellogg's Honey Smacks	5.0
General Mills Nature Valley 100% Natural	4.5
Kellogg's Nut & Honey Crunch O's	4.5
Kellogg's Raisin Bran	4.5
Post Super Golden Crisp	4.0

Cereal	Teaspoons of Sugar per Cup of Cereal
Ralston Real Ghostbusters	4.0
Quaker Cap'n Crunch	4.0

Most of the other popular cereals have at least three teaspoons of sugar per cup of cereal. Here are some no-sugar or *relatively* low-sugar popular cereals:

Cereal	Teaspoons of Sugar per Cup of Cereal
Kellogg's All-Bran	0.0
Nabisco Spoon-Size Shredded Wheat	0.0
General Mills Cheerios	less than 0.5
General Mills Kix	0.5
Kellogg's Corn Flakes	0.5
General Mills Wheaties	1.0
Kellogg's Nutri-Grain Wheat	1.0
Kellogg's Product 19	1.0
Kellogg's Rice Krispies	1.0
Kellogg's Special K	1.0

If you are going to use commercial, packaged cereals, use the ones with the least sugar, as listed above.

Be a Snack Sleuth

Americans spend about $12 billion a year on snacks such as chips, pretzels, pork rinds, popcorn, and cheese puffs. The following figures from the U.S. Department of Agriculture tell you what's in one cup of some popular snacks. (An asterisk indicates a recommended snack, as long as the amount is moderate.)

Food	Calories	Fat (grams)	Sodium (milligrams)
Cheese puffs or twists	236	15	447
Cheddar pretzel	510	21	1,189
*Popcorn, air-popped	31	Trace	0
Popcorn, oil-popped, salt added	55	3	97
Popcorn, caramel-coated, with peanuts	171	3	126
Pork skins, plain	116	7	391
Pork skins, barbecue flavor	114	7	567
Potato chips, plain	152	10	168
Potato chips, barbecue	139	9	213
*Pretzels, without added salt	162	2	123

Food	Calories	Fat (grams)	Sodium (milligrams)
Pretzels, with added salt	162	2	729
*Rice cakes, plain, 1 cake	35	Trace	29
Tortilla chips, plain	178	9	188
Tortilla chips, nacho flavor	176	9	251
Trail mix, with raisins; oil-roasted peanuts, cashews, almonds, pumpkin seed kernels; dried sunflower seed kernels, dates, coconut	693	44	343
Almonds, dry-roasted	810	71	15
Almonds, oil-roasted	970	91	16
Cashews, oil-roasted	748	63	22
Mixed nuts, dry-roasted	814	70	16
Mixed nuts, oil-roasted	876	80	16
Peanuts, oil-roasted, added salt	837	71	624

To add to that list of snacks, here is a short survey of some popular candies. (On the average, each American eats about twenty-one pounds of candy a year.)

Candy	Weight (ounces)	Calories	Fat (grams)
Almond Joy	1.76	250	14
Baby Ruth	2.1	290	14

Candy	Weight (ounces)	Calories	Fat (grams)
Butterfinger	2.1	280	12
Hershey's milk chocolate	1.55	240	14
Junior mints	1.6	192	5
Life Savers (11 candies)	0.9	88	0
M&M's (plain)	1.69	230	10
M&M's (peanut)	1.74	250	13
Milky Way	2.15	280	11
Nestlé Crunch	1.55	220	11
Raisinets	1.58	190	11
Reese's peanut butter cups (2 cups)	1.6	250	15
Snickers (regular flavor)	2.07	280	13
3 Musketeers	2.13	260	9
Tootsie Roll	2.25	252	6
York peppermint pattie	1.5	180	4

85

Time Your Snacks
to Help You

A late afternoon snack is frequently a good idea, especially if you have had an early breakfast and lunch. But avoid after-dinner snacks, especially just before bedtime. The idea is to concentrate on healthy, low-calorie snacks. Here are just a few suggestions:

A piece of fresh fruit
Low-salt salsa with no-salt tortilla chips (see the recipe on page 217)
A plain bagel
Vegetable dips
Nonfat cheese on a low-salt cracker
Chicken-breast slices on a low-salt cracker

You can think of plenty of others.

86

Rely on Relaxation

On a physical level, relaxation improves your circulation and relaxes your muscles. On a higher, mental level, it eases your mind and clears your judgment. Relaxation doesn't necessarily create anything new. Instead, it gives your mind and body a chance to return to their natural, energized states.

Unfortunately, the everyday pressures of life usually don't allow us to relax and rejuvenate ourselves naturally. Strangely enough, relaxation is something we must learn. Few people are ever relaxed enough to fend off the everyday strains that eventually wear them down. Passive relaxation is helpful, but usually only fleeting in its rewards. Something active must be added, and that something for many people is physical activity.

Your mind and body need to be relaxed, and that can be achieved partially by deep breathing and simple meditation. But if relaxation is to have its optimum effect, it must reach deep down into the tired recesses of your body—your spine, your joints, even your cells must be rejuvenated. How is this accomplished? By playing. By running. By walking. By moving.

One of my patients works in the city and used to take taxis to and from his office. After dinner he needed two or three glasses of whiskey to put him to sleep. Now he walks back and forth to work, does not drink after dinner, and has healthy, sound sleep.

He also reduced his weight from 200 to 180 pounds in five months.

There is yet another spoke in the wheel of positive relaxation: a proper, positive, complete diet. You cannot feel good if you eat badly.

87

Know Your Olive Oils

After olives are crushed, releasing much of the oil, the remaining olive paste is *pressed,* an important term to remember when buying olive oil. The first pressing is the least forceful, producing the most desirable *first-pressed* oil. Look for that term or *first cold pressing* on the label. (It might also say *first cold pressed.*) Subsequent pressings are inferior to the first one in quality.

After pressing, the oil is decanted, filtered, settled, and tested for taste and acidity. An oil with less than 1 percent acidity is considered to be "extra-virgin," the prime category (as noted on the label). Olive oil produced in the United States cannot be called "extra-virgin" if it has been chemically processed. If the oil has 1 to 3 percent acidity, it is classified as "virgin."

Extra-virgin olive oil need not be used for cooking, since high heat can destroy its flavor. Its best uses are for salads and other dishes where the flavor of the oil is meant to be dominant. Each brand of olive oil has a distinctive flavor and color. Try a few brands to see which one you like best.

While you are sampling the small sizes of different brands, don't be fooled into thinking that the most expensive one is necessarily the best. Some excellent olive oils are moderately priced. I am looking at a first-rate 34-ounce bottle of first cold pressed, extra-virgin olive oil that costs under seven dollars. Once you choose your favorite brand, you will probably want to buy one of the more economical large sizes.

Store olive oil in a cool, dark, dry place, since it can be damaged by heat, light, or dampness. A properly stored oil should stay fresh for up to a year, but I hope you will use it more frequently than that.

Instead of putting butter or margarine on your French or Italian bread, try dipping the bread in a saucer of olive oil instead. Many fine restaurants are offering small decanters of fresh olive oil as an alternative to butter. A piece of good bread dipped in olive oil is a remarkably delicious treat.

Enhance Your Sexual Activity Sensibly

An increase in sexual activity will not help you lose weight, but weight loss may help you increase your sexual activity. Why?

When it comes to burning off calories, sexual intercourse is no more effective than taking a brisk walk around the block. In fact, it would take about thirteen hours of sexual activity to lose one pound.

How are diet and sex related? Fat people usually have so much sugar in their blood that their sexual interest and performance are decreased. Crash diets almost always impair sexual potency, and they may even create a psychological tension that makes it difficult to achieve sexual pleasure.

If your food intake is adjusted so that blood fats are lowered, it is possible to prevent some physical problems that cause impotence. Most of my patients who are trying to lose weight tell me that one of the fringe benefits of my low-fat, high-complex-carbohydrate eating and activity plan is that they have an increased sexual desire and ability. It seems to be just a question of proper maintenance—just the way a well-tuned car performs better than a badly maintained one.

What about aphrodisiacs and vitamin E? Don't look for "sexy" foods that suddenly turn you into a sexual athlete. No such food exists. Most so-called aphrodisiacs are merely sharp foods that irritate the urogenital tract. Such irritants, whether they are foods or drugs, are potentially harmful, and they certainly are not recommended. The closest thing I ever found to a real sexual stimulant is a sensible program of a well-balanced diet, complemented by physical activity and a relaxed attitude.

Some vitamins, especially E, have also been publicized as enhancers of sexual activity. Vitamin E dilates (enlarges) the blood vessels, and in this way it allows a free flow of blood, which increases the oxygen supply to the body. Physical activity has the same effect and is a lot more reliable. Whatever you do, do not take massive doses of vitamin E, since it tends to accumulate in the body and may have harmful side effects when taken in huge amounts. I recommend 400 I.U. (International Units) a day as a general supplement, not as a sexual enhancer.

Take Care of Your Teeth

Here's a point that is too often ignored: Take care of your teeth and gums. If you can't chew properly, you won't eat properly.

Nowadays, with such excellent dental care available, there is no reason to live with gum disease or tooth loss. If you visit your dentist twice a year, you will be able to *prevent* serious problems from arising.

Have Healthy Snackfests

Before the 1993 Super Bowl, the Snack Food Association and the California Avocado Commission estimated the consumption of specific snacks in the United States on Super Bowl Sunday.

Here are the figures, in *millions of pounds:*

Guacamole	12.0
Potato chips	5.8
Tortilla chips	4.6
Popcorn	3.1
Pretzels	1.5
Nuts	1.5
Cheese puffs	0.9
Corn chips	0.9
Party mix	0.3

Television snacking can be murder, but it doesn't have to be. First of all, let's give the special-event snacker the benefit of the doubt and assume that such voluminous snacking really does happen only once or twice a year. (Thank goodness the Olympics take place only once every two years.)

If such snackfests really are annual events for you, and such an occasion is worth the extra pounds, fine. But most people indulge in television snacking on a more regular basis—the football season, the long cold winter, weekly video movie nights, all day Sunday, and so on. If that's the case, you have to develop better habits. Here are a few suggestions:

1. Put popcorn on the top of your list, as long as it's the air-popped, unsalted, unbuttered variety. This is not really a hardship, with all the excellent ready-to-pop, microwavable "light" popcorns available. They all taste terrific.

2. Buy fruits, vegetables, and a low-fat dip instead of candy and cookies. Before the game begins, cut up a lot of carrots and other raw vegetables to eat by themselves or with the dip.

3. If you are watching the Academy Awards or another night-time event, stop snacking halfway through. You will feel a lot better if you go to bed without a full stomach.

4. If you are watching the Super Bowl or a similar sports event, stop snacking at halftime.

5. Get up and walk around during commercials. It's always a good idea to go to the kitchen for a glass of water.

Bask in a Bubble Bath

Being *aware* of time is not the same as *managing* time, or time management. Time management is a wonderful thing because it allows you to use your time more efficiently, but in the long run what it means is that you are doing twice as much as you did before. Right now, I'm more interested in helping you slow down than speed up.

What I'm asking you to do is to *claim* some time for yourself. People usually set time priorities in this order: (1) work, (2) family, and (3) themselves. You're at the bottom of the list, and you probably feel that's where you should be. Most people feel they can't take time for themselves when there is so much else to do. That's a feeling you should change. The first step should be carving out thirty minutes a day just for yourself. This is your undisturbed, nonproductive time. That doesn't mean you can't share the time with someone you want to be with, as long as the choice is yours.

Maybe you want to read a book without worrying that you should be doing something else, or take a walk just for pleasure instead of thinking of it as exercise, or maybe even work in your garden, where the only thing that matters is that you are *there*. But I've seen people turn thirty minutes in the garden into a stressful time. How? By trying to grow the largest tomatoes in the neighborhood. By producing more roses than their neighbor. By having the perfect lawn. That's not relaxation—that's competition.

Look for activities that envelope you completely, that make you aware only of what you are doing *now*, with no thought about what *else* you might be doing. What good is "nonproductive" time if it makes you feel guilty?

Nonproductive time needs to be ritualized, because a ritual honors a time and a space. When you go into the bathroom, lock the door, and take a bubble bath, you are creating your *private time and space*. It's like taking a nap at just the right time of the day, for just the right amount of time. When you wake up, you feel refreshed and ready to do whatever needs to be done. Your motor is on, but it isn't racing.

A lot of the things we want to do don't happen. Use your nonproductive time to let them happen. Make time for yourself.

92

Shop for Food
When You're Not Hungry

Many people can shop only after work, when they are hungry and too tired to stop and read food labels. If you shop when you are hungry you will buy extra food—and once you buy it, you will eat it. Often, working people open their packages and nibble on their food before they even get to the checkout counter.

If you have a choice, shop right after breakfast, lunch, or dinner. If you work all day and you *must* shop on your way home from work, try to eat a piece of fruit just before you leave your office to help stave off your hunger, and then make a conscious effort not to buy more than you need.

93 ◇ Check Out Cross-Training

The concept called "cross-training" became popular in the early 1980s, and its popularity continues today. The idea of cross-training is to combine several different physical activities. The triathlon competition (swimming, biking, and running) is one form of cross-training, developed when running alone did not seem to fulfill the needs of many fitness buffs.

Since not everyone is fit enough to be a triathlete, runners also began playing basketball, tennis, or other sports along with their running. Some other activities that can be combined with running or walking are aerobic dancing, stationary biking or rowing, weight lifting, and stair climbing. Cross-training relieves the constant pressure on the same muscles every day, resting muscles and preventing injury; it relieves boredom; and it promotes better overall fitness, encouraging weight loss and toning specific muscle groups of your choice.

If you decide to try cross-training (it is not recommended for everyone), be realistic about it. Don't expect too much from yourself too soon. Remember: Physical activity should be fun, not torture. I totally disagree with the phrase "No pain, no gain." If there's pain, stop.

Eat More
Omega-3 Fatty Acids

Omega-3 fatty acids are polyunsaturated fats found mostly in fish such as salmon, bluefish, whitefish, swordfish, rainbow trout, striped bass, and squid. They can also be obtained from plants that contain linolenic acid. Such plants and plant derivatives include linseed oil, walnuts, flaxseed, canola oil, soybeans, spinach, and mustard greens. The linolenic acid in these plants is converted in your body into omega-3 fatty acids.

The benefits of omega-3 fatty acids are being reconfirmed after a brief period of popularity in the 1980s. Studies show that omega-3 fatty acids help reduce the incidence of high blood pressure, high triglyceride levels, low blood-clotting times, cancer, and inflammatory diseases such as arthritis. Also, the omega-3 fatty acids found in breast milk are essential for the proper development of vision and of the brain in newborns.

The optimal intake of omega-3s is about 0.8 to 1.1 grams a day. These amounts can be achieved by eating the recommended fish two or three times a week. Too much omega-3 fatty acid can cause a deficient immune system and brain hemorrhaging, so please don't overdo it. Fish-oil supplements are not a good idea because they are so concentrated that they may cause an overdose. As usual, rely on a well-balanced diet for your nutritional needs.

Stay Physically Fit
throughout Your Life

More and more schools are eliminating physical education classes as a way of cutting expenses. That's a foolhardy notion. If children are taught that physical activity is not important, it's a lesson they will never forget. And we'll lose money in the long run: inactive children tend to become inactive, overweight adults, costing society a fortune in health-care benefits.

About 60 percent of American adults lead sedentary lives. We may think we're more active than we used to be, but it's just not true. I know plenty of people who join a physical fitness club but are never there, or who buy fitness machines that they don't use. Almost a third of Americans get *no* exercise. In fact, according to the Centers for Disease Control, only 22 percent of Americans are physically active to levels recommended for good health.

A panel of doctors and fitness experts in the United States convened in the spring of 1993 to formulate recommendations about promoting lifelong physical activity. The panel encouraged schools, employers, and community groups to keep playgrounds and gymnasiums open, develop more accessible walking paths and parks, provide exercise rooms and equipment, and encourage walking and bicycling for transportation.

Face the Truth
about Fast Foods

In 1986 it was made public that fast-food chains such as McDonald's, Burger King, Wendy's, Arby's, and Big Boy were cooking their food in beef tallow, a highly saturated form of fat. Some chains were using palm oil, which is even more heavily saturated than beef tallow. To their credit, most of the chains have stopped using beef tallow and have taken other measures to reduce the amount of fat in their foods. But as you will see in the following lists, even the foods with the least amounts of fat still have a lot. For example, Burger King's broiler chicken sandwich is their lowest-fat food (not counting salads), but it still contains 18 grams of fat. However, that is a tremendous improvement over their highest-fat food, a double Whopper hamburger with cheese, which contains 61 grams of fat.

As an instant guide to fast-food from chains, here are the best picks from well-known chains, as of May 1991:

1. McDonald's McLean Deluxe sandwich: 320 calories, 10 grams fat.

2. Burger King broiler chicken sandwich: 379 calories, 18 grams fat.

3. Wendy's grilled chicken sandwich: 340 calories, 13 grams fat.

4. Kentucky Fried Chicken Lite 'n Crispy drumsticks (two): 242 calories, 14 grams fat.

The *real* best picks at fast-food restaurants are the salads and baked potatoes that most chains now serve. Pick a low-fat dressing for your salad, preferably oil and vinegar.

And here are the *worst* fast-food picks:

1. McDonald's Filet-O-Fish sandwich: 440 calories, 26 grams fat. (The excellent qualities of fish can be ruined in its preparation.)

2. Burger King Double Whopper with cheese: 935 calories, 61 grams fat.

3. Wendy's Big Classic: 570 calories, 33 grams fat.

4. Kentucky Fried Chicken sandwich: 482 calories, 27 grams fat. (Chicken, too, can be cooked in such a way that it becomes undesirable.)

Although most fast-food chains have tried to conform to the latest nutritional guidelines, the public has not always followed suit. Many people now buy two hamburgers instead of one because the hamburgers are reduced in fat and calories, with the result being too many calories and too much fat. Don't forget that Burger King's best still gives you 36 grams of fat, and that doesn't count the fat in french fries and a milkshake.

Take Food with You
When You Travel

Travel has gotten so annoying and full of hassles, one of which is having nothing good to eat. Whether it's airplane chicken or snacks from roadside vending machines, you can usually expect a long day of travel with nothing decent to eat.

Every year Americans take over a billion trips. Eating well might seem to be a problem if you're in your car all day, but it need not be. When my wife and I take a long car ride, we always carry along a loaf of fresh whole-grain bread, water, a couple of pieces of fresh fruit, and knives, forks, spoons, and napkins. If we want to stop to eat something, we are not tempted by the many fast-food chains along the way. Instead, we drive into the closest town and stop at a food market, where we buy fresh tomatoes or low-fat cheese to eat with our bread.

For dessert, we usually buy fresh fruit in season, which often includes melon, an excellent choice all the way around. Cantaloupe contains significant amounts of beta-carotene, vitamins A and C, folic acid, and fiber. Half a cantaloupe contains only about 60 calories, and it tastes so good. And don't forget the honeydew and watermelon—and berries, which contain more fiber than a slice of bread and have a fair amount of vitamin C.

How to turn heads on an airplane? Peel an orange—all eyes will turn to the fresh smell, the unexpected thrill of *fresh food.* Also, it gives you the pleasure (sorely needed when traveling) of feeling that you are *in control.*

Focus on the Special
Things You Can Do

For many years John Wooden was the coach of the UCLA basket-ball team. He was known as a man who knew how to win, but he was also known as a true gentleman and a positive thinker. He once said, "Don't let what you cannot do interfere with what you can do." His comment reminds us that our capabilities are much more important than our limitations.

Everyone has limitations. The great Roman poet Virgil said, "We cannot do all things." We would be foolish to think we could. But just because you can't build a bookcase or fly a jet airplane doesn't mean you are a failure. Think of all the things you *can* do. In fact, go one step further. Think of that very special gift you have for doing something *better* than almost anyone else. You are unique. Don't forget it.

John Wooden's basketball teams won the national champion-ship eight times between 1964 and 1975. During that time they won the championship seven years in a row; no other college team has ever won it more than twice in a row. Wooden's teams were a plea-sure to watch. Every year he would have a new team to deal with, and every year you could see that he had made a change here and another one there to accommodate his new players' talents. This year's team may not have been as good as last year's, but Wooden's teams won anyway. Instead of just trying to win, his players *expected* to win. And they did.

One of my patients had an interesting career change because she realized what she could do and what she couldn't do. All her life she had wanted to be a writer, but despite the finest education and dedication to that craft, one rejection followed another. Her husband was already an established writer, and he noticed that she always made important suggestions about his work that she seemed unable to see in her own work. He suggested that maybe she was a better editor than a writer—no disgrace, since really good editors are rare. After her initial resistance, she decided to look around and see what the possibilities were for entering publishing as an editor instead of a writer. It took a few years to get started, but today she is one of the top editors in the country, if not the world.

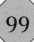

Go for the "Good" Cholesterol

High-density lipoproteins (HDLs), are commonly called the "good" cholesterol because they lower the risk of cardiovascular disease by removing plaque from the inside of blood vessels and they may help fight infections. HDLs may be increased in your body by eating a low-fat diet, including monounsaturated fats such as olive oil and canola oil, but there are other ways also.

When people lose weight, they usually increase their level of HDLs while decreasing their level of LDLs (low-density lipoproteins, the "bad" cholesterol). Even moderate exercise will help lower your LDL level, while aerobic exercise will help boost your HDL level. It is estimated that a year of regular brisk walking can raise your HDL level more than 25 percent. Postmenopausal women who are receiving estrogen replacement therapy usually get the extra benefit of a higher HDL level and a lower LDL level. Also, smokers can raise their HDL level by quitting their habit. The two most important factors in raising your level of HDLs are regular physical activity and a low-fat diet.

Affirm Life-Enhancing Values

The world seems to be rushing past us so fast that it is becoming more and more difficult to remember who we are and what we stand for. But when everything else is falling apart around us, we have to know precisely what our values are. Some days, when nothing and no one seems to make sense, when our politicians, our bankers, our doctors, and even our clergy have failed us, we may be left with *only* our values, and those values keep us from being alone and unprotected.

What *does* hold us together when the outside world seems so chaotic? Our families. Our belief in our work. And our values.

Two goals of a full and rewarding life should be (1) to find your own identity, and (2) to express your unique talents with as little stress as possible. But our goals, conscious and unconscious, short-term and long-term, must go beyond that. In order for you to lead a happy, relaxed, and satisfying life, you must *give something of the best of yourself to others.*

We are social animals, no less than ants or honeybees, although we certainly have more to say about our choices than they do. But like ants and honeybees, we cannot live alone. A honeybee alone is nothing; it has no purpose. In a sense, it is not even a bee, since it is not doing the things that bees normally do. Maybe a person alone, without sharing his or her innate gifts, is not even a person.

A FEW GUIDELINES

Useful Tables
Vitamins and Minerals: Are You Getting Enough?
How to Read Food Labels

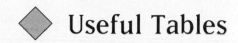 # Useful Tables

---

FOODS TO AVOID MOST OF THE TIME

Anchovies

Avocados

Beer (light beer OK)

Butter

Cake

Catsup

Coleslaw

Cold cuts

Cookies

Cream

Custard

Dried apricots

Frankfurters

Hamburgers

Honey

Jams and jellies (low-sugar OK)

Nuts

Pastries

Pickles

Pies

Prepared salad dressing

Pudding

Raisins

Salt (including sea salt)

Smoked fish

Soy sauce

Sugar

Whole milk, whole yogurt

FOODS YOU MAY BE AVOIDING UNNECESSARILY

Bagels, salt-free, egg-free
Bread, whole-grain, low-salt
   French, Italian, pita
Breadsticks, no salt
Cheese, low-fat, low-salt
Dips, homemade
Fresh-fruit popsicles
Matzoh

Oatmeal
Pancakes or waffles, without
   butter or syrup
Pasta
Popcorn, air-popped, without
   salt or butter
Potatoes, not fried
Rice

FOODS TO EAT REGULARLY

Bread, whole-grain
Cereal, whole-grain, including
   rice, Wheatena, farina,
   oatmeal, grits, buckwheat,
   kasha, couscous
Chicken, white, skinless
Cottage cheese, low-fat, low-salt
Fish, unsmoked
Fruit, fresh
Herbs and spices, especially in
   place of salt
Juice, fresh or frozen (add low-
   salt seltzer if you want a
   carbonated drink)

Pasta, without cream sauce
Potatoes, not fried
Safflower, corn, canola, or
   olive oil
Salads, with vinaigrette or
   other low-fat dressing
Turkey, white, skinless
Tuna, water-packed
Vegetables, fresh or frozen,
   preferably fresh
Water, 6–8 glasses a day,
   preferably not with meals

Meat: 4 ounces, cooked, without bone or fat

Fish: 4 ounces, cooked, without bone or skin

Poultry: 4 ounces, cooked, without bone, fat, or skin

Vegetable (other than potato): 1/2 cup

Fruit: 1 whole fruit, except 1/2 grapefruit, 1/2 small cantaloupe
    or 1/4 large cantaloupe, 1/4 honeydew melon

Juice: 4 ounces

Skim milk, low-fat milk, buttermilk: 1 cup (8 ounces)

Bread: 2 slices

Cooked cereal: 1/3 cup, uncooked

Prepared cereal: 1 cup

Whole-grain food: 1/4 cup uncooked, 1/2 cup cooked

Pasta: 2 ounces (or 1/2 cup cooked)

Matzoh: 1/2 to 1 board

Vegetable oil: 1 tablespoon

Low-fat cottage cheese: 1/2 cup

Low-fat yogurt: 1/2 cup

Potato: small to medium

Meat (4 ounces, cooked, well trimmed)	Fat (grams)
Bacon, 3 strips	9
Beef frankfurter, cured	32
Bologna, 1 slice	6
Brisket, trimmed, braised	14
Chicken breast, skinless	5
Chicken breast, with skin	9
Chicken wing, with skin	22
Duck, skinless	10
Duck, with skin	32
Eye of round, select	7
Ground beef, broiled	21
Leg of lamb	9
Liver, pan fried	9
Pork tenderloin	6
Salami	24
Sausage, Italian	31
Veal, shoulder roast	8
Sirloin, trimmed, broiled	10
T-bone steak, trimmed, broiled	12
Tenderloin, select	11
Turkey breast, skinless	1
Turkey breast, with skin	3

Compare the fat grams in this table with those in the following one. The message is clear, isn't it?

FAT CONTENT IN VEGETABLES

Vegetable	Fat (grams)
Asparagus, cooked, 4 spears	0
Avocado, 1 medium	30
Beans, cooked, 1 cup	1
Beets, cooked, 1 cup	0
Broccoli, cooked, 1 cup	0
Brussels sprouts, cooked, 1 cup	1
Cabbage, raw, 1 cup	0
Cauliflower, cooked, 1 cup	0
Celery, raw, 1 stalk	0
Corn, cooked, 1 cup	0
Cucumber, raw, 1	0
Eggplant, cooked, 1 cup	0
Lentils, cooked, 1 cup	1
Mushrooms, raw, 1 cup	0
Onions, chopped, 1/4 cup	0
Peas, cooked, 1 cup	0
Pepper, sweet, raw	0
Potato, baked with skin	0
Potato, fried in vegetable oil, 2 ounces	8
Potato, mashed, with milk and margarine, 1 cup	9
Soybeans, cooked, 1 cup	10
Spinach, raw, 1 cup	0
Split peas, cooked, 1 cup	1
String beans, cooked, 1 cup	0
Sweet potato, baked	0
Tofu, 4 ounces	5
Tomatoes, canned, 1 cup	1
Tomato, raw, 1	0

FAT CONTENT IN FISH AND SHELLFISH

Food (4 ounces, cooked, except caviar)	Fat (grams)
Carp	8
Caviar, 2 tablespoons	6
Clams	2
Clams, breaded, fried	13
Cod	1
Crab, Alaskan king	2
Crayfish	1
Haddock	1
Halibut	3
Lobster	1
Mackerel	21
Mussels	5
Oysters	6
Perch	1
Pike	1
Salmon, pink, canned	7
Salmon, sockeye, fresh	13
Sardines, canned in oil, with bones	13
Scallops	1
Scallops, breaded, fried	14
Shrimp	1
Shrimp, breaded, fried	14
Snapper	2
Squid, fried	8
Swordfish	6
Trout, rainbow	5
Tuna, light, water-packed	2
Tuna, light, oil-packed	9
Tuna, bluefin, fresh	7

FAT CONTENT IN NUTS

Nut	Fat (grams)
Almonds, 1 ounce	15
Cashews, dry roasted, 1 ounce	13
Chestnuts, roasted, 1 ounce	1
Coconut, dried, sweetened, 1 ounce	10
Hazelnuts, 1 ounce	18
Macadamia nuts, roasted in oil, 1 ounce	22
Peanuts, roasted in oil, 1 ounce	14
Pecans, 1 ounce	19
Pistachios, 1 ounce	14
Sesame seeds, 1 tablespoon	4
Sunflower seeds, 1 ounce	14
Walnuts, 1 ounce	16

FAT CONTENT IN SOME SWEETS

Food	*Fat (grams)*
Angel food cake, 2-ounce slice	0
Caramels, 1 ounce	3
Carrot cake, with cream cheese frosting, 2-ounce slice	12
Cheesecake, 2-ounce slice	11
Chocolate, with almonds, 1 ounce	10
Chocolate-chip cookies, 4 small	11
Chocolate pudding, $1/2$ cup	4
Coffee cake, 2-ounce slice	5
Devil's food cake, with chocolate frosting, 2-ounce slice	6
Fig bars, 4	4
Fudge, 1 ounce	3
Ice cream, $1/2$ cup	7
Ice milk, $1/2$ cup	3
Jelly beans, 1 ounce	0
Marshmallows, 1 ounce	0
Oatmeal-raisin cookies, 4	10
Peanut butter cookies, 4	14
Pie, 2-ounce slice	6–13
Popsicle, fruit or juice	0
Rice pudding, $1/2$ cup	4
Sherbet, $1/2$ cup	2
Sorbet, $1/2$ cup	0
Shortbread cookies, 4	8
Tapioca pudding, $1/2$ cup	4
Vanilla wafers, 4	3

FAT CONTENT IN SOME FAST FOODS AND SNACK FOODS

Food	*Fat (grams)*
Cheese puffs, 1 ounce	10
Cheeseburger, plain, on bun	15
Cheeseburger, double-decker, with condiments	35
Chicken, fried, dark meat, 2 pieces	27
English muffin, with egg, cheese, bacon	20
Fish sandwich, with tartar sauce	23
French fries, fried in vegetable oil	12
Hamburger, plain, on bun	12
Pancakes, with butter and syrup	14
Pizza, cheese, 1 slice	3
Popcorn, air-popped, plain, 1 cup	0
Popcorn, oil-popped, with butter, 1 cup	15
Potato, baked, with cheese sauce	21
Potato chips, 1 ounce	10
Pretzels, 1 ounce (8 pretzels)	1
Roast beef sandwich, plain	14
Salad, tossed, with chicken	4
Tortilla chips, 1 ounce	8

Instead of	Substitute	Fat grams Saved
Bacon, cooked, 1 ounce	Canadian bacon, cooked, 1 ounce	12
Beef tenderloin, choice, untrimmed, broiled, 4 ounces	Beef tenderloin, select, trimmed, broiled, 4 ounces	11
Corn chips, 1 ounce	Air-popped popcorn, plain, 1 ounce	9
Cream cheese, 1 ounce	Cottage cheese, low-fat, 1 ounce	9
Croissant	Bagel, plain	10
Fast-food french fries, regular serving size	Baked potato, medium	11
Hard salami, 1 ounce	Extra-lean roasted ham, 1 ounce	8
Ice cream, premium, 1 cup	Sorbet, 1 cup	24
Lamp chop, untrimmed, broiled, 4 ounces	Lean leg of lamb, trimmed, broiled, 4 ounces	32
Oil-packed light tuna, 4 ounces	Water-packed light tuna, 4 ounces	7
Oil-roasted peanuts, 1 ounce	Roasted chestnuts, 1 ounce	13

Instead of	Substitute	Fat grams Saved
Pork spareribs, cooked, 4 ounces	Lean pork loin, trimmed, broiled, 4 ounces	18
Potato chips, 1 ounce	Thin pretzels, 1 ounce (8 pretzels)	9
Roast duck, skinless, 4 ounces	Roast chicken, skinless, 4 ounces	8
Whole egg	Egg white	6

◆ Vitamins and Minerals: Are You Getting Enough?

Because so many people are on one "diet" or another, I wanted to talk a little about the possible need for vitamin and mineral dietary supplements. A word of caution at the outset: *Don't exceed my dosage suggestions.* (Two is not always better than one.) Overdoses of vitamins and minerals can be harmful.

Of course, my first choice is always that you eat three well-balanced meals a day, but for many people that is becoming less and less realistic. So vitamin and mineral supplements are more important than ever to ensure that you get all the nutrients you need. Vitamins and minerals *alone* cannot take the place of a regular, well-balanced diet. Also, megadoses of vitamins interfere with the absorption of food nutrients.

Remember: Vitamin and mineral supplements are *not a substitute* for a well-balanced diet.

VITAMINS

Vitamins are chemical compounds that your body needs in small amounts to help regulate metabolism. They always contain carbon. Vitamins A, D, E, and K are usually classified as *fat-soluble* vitamins, which can be stored in the body for relatively long periods. Vitamin C and the B vitamins are *water soluble* and are stored in the body for only a day or two. Water-soluble vitamins are often lost during cooking because they dissolve in the cooking water or are degraded by heat. Vitamin deficiencies can cause many different disorders.

Vitamins that are present in foods are called *natural.* Those that are created in the laboratory are called *synthetic.* Chemically, there is no difference between natural and synthetic vitamins. Synthetic vitamins are less expensive, however, and can usually be kept fresher longer than natural vitamins can.

As you probably know already, clear-cut information about the benefits of vitamin supplements has been difficult to find in the past. But now it seems that researchers are agreeing (at least more than they used to) about the need to supplement our daily diets. The overall conclusion is this: Relatively large doses of some vitamins may help prevent diseases such as cancer and cardiovascular disease, and some may also ease the aging process.

Check the expiration dates on vitamin labels. If the vitamins expire in less than nine months, don't buy them. Manufacturers are allowed to choose their own expiration dates, and the vitamins may have been bottled for several years.

VITAMIN A. Usually there is no need to take supplements of vitamin A, especially because excessive doses tend to build up in toxic amounts. Vitamin A is not water soluble. Main food sources: liver, egg yolks, whole milk, butter.

BETA-CAROTENE. Beta-carotene is a previtamin that your body converts into vitamin A; however, beta-carotene is a more efficient antioxidant than vitamin A. (An *antioxidant* is a substance that helps eliminate the harmful by-products that occur when cells use oxygen to "burn" their fuel. Oxidants are also known as free radicals.) Like vitamin A, beta-carotene is not water soluble. I recommend 10,000 I.U. (International Units) a day. The combination of beta-carotene and 500 micrograms of selenium is a powerful cancer preventive; selenium is found mainly in seafood. Main food sources of beta-carotene: carrots, leafy green vegetables, yellow and orange vegetables, fruits, liver, egg yolks, dairy products, oils.

B VITAMINS. Take a B-complex vitamin supplement with at least 100 milligrams each of the B vitamins. The B vitamins include B_1 (thiamine), B_2 (riboflavin), B_6 (pyridoxine), B_{12} (cyanocobalamin), biotin, folic acid (B_9), inositol, niacin (B_3), and pantothenic acid (B_5). The B vitamins are water soluble. Food sources of vitamin B include whole grains, vegetables, and fish.

VITAMIN C. I recommend a maximum daily supplement of vitamin C of 2 to 3 grams (2,000 to 3,000 milligrams). Use calcium ascorbate or ascorbic acid, but not sodium ascorbate, which contains too much sodium. A 1993 study at Arizona State University showed that 2,000 milligrams of vitamin C a day reduced the histamine level in the body by 40 percent. (Excess histamine interferes with the proper functioning of the immune system; it is what "antihistamines" counteract.) Vitamin C is water soluble. Main food sources: citrus fruits, butter, tomatoes, green peppers, sweet red peppers, broccoli, potatoes, raw cabbage.

VITAMIN D. There is usually no need for a daily supplement of vitamin D, especially because it is not water soluble and it can have toxic buildups. The elderly should increase their intake of dietary vitamin D, since it helps prevent or minimize osteoporosis, and some postmenopausal women may need to consider hormonal supplements as well. Main food sources: fish oils, liver, milk, egg yolk, butter. Vitamin D is also synthesized by your body when your skin is exposed to sunlight.

VITAMIN E. Take 400 I.U. of vitamin E daily, but not with vitamin B, since some B vitamins contain iron, which decreases the effectiveness of vitamin E. Vitamin E is an antioxidant, and it may also help prevent lung cancer. Vitamin E is not water soluble. Main food sources: leafy green vegetables, wheat germ oil, liver, peanuts, eggs.

VITAMIN K. There is usually no need for a dietary supplement of vitamin K, which is not water soluble. Main food sources: yogurt, molasses, safflower oil, liver, leafy green vegetables. Vitamin K is also synthesized in the body by intestinal bacteria.

MINERALS

Minerals are naturally occurring inorganic elements (they do not contain carbon) that are needed for the regulation of metabolism. Some minerals, such as iodine, copper, zinc, cobalt, iron, and manganese, are needed by the body in such small amounts (less than 100 milligrams a day) that they are called *microminerals* or *trace elements*. Calcium, chlorine (chloride), magnesium, phosphorus, potassium, sodium, and sulfur are known as *macrominerals* because they are found in the body in significant amounts.

As with vitamins, there is no need to spend extra money on minerals by buying them in health-food stores.

CALCIUM. Calcium is the most abundant mineral in the body.

Young women, the elderly, and cigarette smokers may need a dietary supplement. Main food sources: dairy products, eggs, fish, soybeans.

CHLORIDE. Athletes and workers who participate in vigorous physical activities may need additional chloride. Main food sources: all foods, table salt.

CHROMIUM. About 200 to 400 micrograms of chromium a day can raise the level of HDLs (the "good" cholesterol) in your blood. Main food sources: meats, vegetables, yeast, beer, unrefined wheat flour, corn oil, shellfish.

MAGNESIUM. Magnesium is important for normal muscle contractions and the conduction of nerve impulses, and it strengthens bones and tooth enamel. Also, it aids the metabolism of calcium and thus helps prevent osteoporosis. Main food sources: green vegetables, milk, meats, nuts.

PHOSPHORUS. Phosphorus deficiencies, which cause rickets (a condition marked by soft, deformed bones), are rare. Main food sources: dairy products, meats, fish, poultry, beans, grains, eggs.

POTASSIUM. Bananas are one of the best sources of potassium, which is important for proper muscle contraction and heartbeat. Other food sources: all foods, especially meats, vegetables, milk.

SELENIUM. As noted earlier, the combination of beta-carotene and 500 micrograms of selenium each day may help prevent cancer. It is difficult to estimate the amount of selenium in foods because different types of soil contain widely varying amounts of selenium. Main food sources: most foods, especially seafood, liver, other meats.

SODIUM. With all the natural sodium in most foods and the added sodium in processed foods, it is virtually impossible to have a sodium deficiency. Remember that sea salt is the same as regular table salt and offers no special benefits. Main food sources: most foods, table salt.

SULFUR. Ordinarily, no dietary supplement of sulfur is necessary. Main food sources: all protein-containing foods.

ZINC. Among other things, zinc may help prevent prostate cancer. Zinc deficiencies are common, and I recommend 25 milligrams a day. Main food sources: meats, liver, seafood, eggs, legumes, milk, green vegetables.

Garlic and Onions
Patient histories show that garlic and onions lower cholesterol levels and help prevent stomach cancer, hypertension, and cardio-vascular disease by detoxifying carcinogens. Cook with fresh garlic and onions, and use fresh garlic in salads; don't use a garlic press, which tends to lose too much of the valuable oil.

FEDERAL RECOMMENDED DOSAGES OF VITAMINS AND MINERALS

A 1992 proposal by the Food and Drug Administration (FDA) would replace the current U.S. Recommended Daily Allowances (RDAs) for vitamins and minerals with a new standard called the Reference Daily Intake (RDI). Rather than increasing the daily intake of vitamins and minerals, as you might expect, the new FDA recommendations would decrease daily intake.

The present RDA system is designed for people of specific age and sex, such as elderly women, while the proposed RDI system concentrates on the dietary needs of average healthy people. Because the RDI system addresses averages only, it could cause confusion, as well as a lower-than-necessary intake of vitamins and minerals. For example, the RDA for calcium is based on the requirements of those who need it most—young women. With the reduced levels of calcium indicated in the RDIs, young women and others in need of high levels of dietary calcium (for example, cigarette smokers and the elderly) would have to be knowledgeable enough to supplement their diets.

SOME EXCEPTIONAL SITUATIONS

Daily vitamin or mineral supplements may be necessary in unusual situations such as the following:

1. Some vegetarians may need supplements of vitamin B12, calcium, iron, and zinc. Check with your physician. About 70 percent of vegetarians take vitamin and mineral supplements.

2. Women with an excessive menstrual flow may need iron supplements.

3. People who consume very few calories (including anorexics, bulimics, and abusers of drugs or alcohol) may need vitamin and mineral supplements to fulfill their daily dietary requirements.

4. Pregnant or breast-feeding women may need extra iron, calcium, and folic acid. Check with your physician.

5. Some diseases and medications tend to disrupt the digestion and absorption of certain nutrients. As a result, you may need vitamin and mineral supplements. Your physician will know when such a situation exists.

6. Smokers should take supplements of vitamin C, vitamin E, vitamin A, beta-carotene, and folic acid.

7. Postmenopausal women should take 400 I.U. of vitamin D, especially if they do not spend a lot of time in the sun.

How to Read Food Labels

We all know that we are supposed to be eating less fat, sugar, sodium, and red meat, while increasing our intake of fiber-rich foods, whole grains, and vegetables. But when we look at a food label, we can't seem to make sense of which foods contain what, or how much, of any given nutrient. In 1990, the Nutritional Labeling and Education Act, which requires understandable labels on food, was passed. However, food labeling is still in the process of being changed, and until food labels actually *do* become understandable, here is some information that may help you read labels easily and accurately.

WHAT DO THE FDA AND THE USDA DO?

The FDA (Food and Drug Administration) checks the safety of foods, drugs, and beverages and the accuracy of their labels. It is not responsible for the regulation of meat, poultry, or alcohol. The USDA (U.S. Department of Agriculture) checks the safety of meats, poultry, and products that contain more than 2 percent poultry and 3 percent meat by weight. The safety of alcoholic beverages is checked by the Bureau of Alcohol, Tobacco, and Firearms, a branch of the Treasury Department.

WHAT'S IN THERE ANYWAY?

Ingredients are listed in the order of highest weight. In the case of Kellogg's Rice Krispies (a random choice) the ingredients are rice, sugar, salt, corn syrup (a sweetener), and malt flavoring. Some prepared breakfast cereals actually begin the list of ingredients with sugar—for example, Quaker Cap'n Crunch's Crunch Berries, Kellogg's Honey Smacks, General Mills Cocoa Puffs, and Post Super Golden Crisp.

If you are checking the amount of sugar in a product, remember that honey, corn syrup, fructose, and other sweeteners may be listed in addition to sugar. All sweeteners should be added together to find the relative amount of sugar in a food.

WHAT IS A "SERVING"?

When a manufacturer states that a product contains 50 calories per serving, the question is, What is a serving? Usually, the manufacturer thinks it's a lot smaller than you do, and you probably eat two or three "servings" as one serving.

It can be even more confusing. A can of diet Coke or diet Pepsi, for instance, turns out to be *two* servings. So in order to get only the 1 calorie advertised, you have to drink only half a can. In other words, you think you are getting 1 calorie because that's what the advertising says, but as you will see, you can't always take an advertisement literally.

Here are some other interesting interpretations of a "serving." Ocean Spray has small containers of fruit drinks that contain 8.45 ounces—a realistic serving size. But according to Ocean Spray, a serving equals only 6 ounces. So what do you do with the leftover

2.45 ounces? With Bachman Thin 'n Light pretzels, a serving is one ounce. But how many *pretzels* is that? (It turns out to be eight pretzels, but who's going to weigh pretzels?) Finally, Entenmann's chocolate loaf cake contains 70 calories per serving, but the serving size is 1 ounce; it would be very difficult to *cut* a 1-ounce piece of cake, let alone accept it as a serving.

WHAT DOES THAT MEAN?

Many of the terms we see on food labels are like "mystery terms," either having confusing meanings or having several different meanings. For example, what do *enriched*, *fortified*, and *no sugar added* mean? Here are the proper definitions of some mystery terms:

CALORIES: The number of calories *per serving*.

DAILY VALUE: The recommended daily amount of protein, vitamins, and minerals. As noted earlier, such an amount used to be called the RDA, or Recommended Daily Allowance.

DIETARY SUPPLEMENT: A product with enough added nutrients in one serving to provide 50 percent of the RDA of vitamins and minerals.

ENRICHED: Contains added nutrients to replace the ones lost in processing.

EXPIRATION DATE: The date a manufacturer suggests is the latest date when freshness can be expected. Because elderly people often rely on packaged and canned foods, they especially need to be aware of expiration dates and other clues about freshness. Unfortunately, our senses of taste and smell become less efficient as we get older, and we might not always be able to detect stale or spoiled food. No matter what age you are, it's a good idea to shop at least once a week and buy food in small quantities to maximize freshness.

FORTIFIED: Contains added nutrients, making those nutrients 10 percent or more of the RDA.

FRESH: Foods labeled "fresh" cannot have been frozen, processed, heated, or preserved chemically.

FROM CONCENTRATE: The water is taken out before the food is shipped, and it is replaced when the food reaches its packaging destination; probably seen most often on juice containers.

HIGH (PROTEIN, FIBER, ETC.): The term *high* means that the food contains at least 10 percent more of the nutrient's RDA than similar products. No regulations exist to regulate how much fiber is "high fiber."

LIGHT OR LITE: A food that derives more than half its calories from fat cannot be called "light" unless it is being compared to a product that has at least 50 percent more fat than it does. *Light* or *lite* can also refer to sodium, calories, or breading, which will be specified on the label. "Light beer" can refer to color, calories, flavor, or alcoholic content, none of which needs to be specified, except calories.

LOW-CALORIE: Contains a maximum of 40 calories per serving; check the size of the serving to see if it's realistic.

LOW-FAT: Food that is lower in fat than the regular food, but not necessarily low in fat.

NATURAL: "Natural" meat and poultry foods have undergone no more than minimal processing and contain no artificial ingredients. Otherwise, *natural* is an unregulated term and means different things to different people. The "Natural" in Mrs. Smith's Natural Juice apple pie refers to the fruit juices used to make the pie; the pie itself contains artificial preservatives.

NATURALLY SWEETENED: Usually means that the product has been sweetened with fruit or juice instead of sugar, but the FDA has no control over this label.

NO ADDITIVES OR PRESERVATIVES: Contains no products designed to enhance nutritional quality; preserve freshness; improve texture, moisture, or consistency; or improve flavor or appearance. The FDA has approved some additives and preservatives that are necessary to preserve the quality of packaged foods, but not all preservatives have been rated as safe by the FDA.

NO CHOLESTEROL; CHOLESTEROL-FREE: This should be self-explanatory—a food either contains cholesterol or it doesn't—but there's an additional wrinkle. Several vegetable oils that never contained cholesterol in the first place (such as Mazola corn oil and HeartBeat canola oil) are now proclaiming that they are cholesterol free; the FDA has ordered that these foods remove their "no-cholesterol" labels. A food may be cholesterol free and still raise your cholesterol level. Such products contain coconut oil, palm oil, or palm kernel oil, all of which contain highly saturated fat.

NO SALT ADDED; UNSALTED: No salt added in processing; contains only the naturally occurring sodium in the food itself, which may be high.

NO SUGAR ADDED; SUGAR-FREE: Contains no sucrose (table sugar), but may contain other sweeteners such as corn syrup or honey, which have little or no nutritional value but *do* contain calories.

PARTIALLY HYDROGENATED: Food containing fat that is 5 to 60 percent saturated.

PRIME BEEF: The most tender cuts, usually because they contain the most fat; the leanest beef is labeled "select." It should be noted that meat does not have to contain any labels at all regarding its fat content, so it is possible that unlabeled beef can be prime or select. Look at the meat itself.

REDUCED CALORIES: Has at least 40 fewer calories per serving than the regular food; some "regular foods" have 400 to 500 calories, however, leaving some reduced-calorie foods high in calories.

REDUCED FAT: Fat reduced by more than 3 grams per serving.

REDUCED SODIUM: Sodium content reduced by 140 milligrams, which is not much. Check the total amount of sodium.

SIGNIFICANT SOURCE OF A NUTRIENT: Provides at least 10 percent of the RDA for that nutrient.

SODIUM-FREE: Less than 5 milligrams of sodium per serving.

UNSWEETENED: The product does not contain added sugar.

SOME MISLEADING CLAIMS

Here's an example of the kind of misleading double standard that the federal regulations hope to eliminate: Monosodium glutamate (MSG) must be listed on the label, because some people are allergic to it. But hydrogenated vegetable protein may be listed as "natural flavoring," even though it contains MSG.

When fat is listed by weight, it sounds a lot better than when it is listed by calories, because fat is very light. A label may say a food contains only 20 percent fat, but that 20 percent may account for 75 percent or more of the food's calorie content. In other words (as if you didn't know), fat is fattening.

You may see a label that includes "soybean and/or coconut oil" in its ingredients. The manufacturer doesn't have to specify which oil was used, even though soybean oil is polyunsaturated and coconut oil is saturated.

The term *carbohydrates* on the label includes sugar, fiber, and complex carbohydrates. The specific types of carbohydrates may or may not be listed separately.

Specific food colors and flavors do not have to be listed on the label, except for Yellow No. 5, which causes an allergic reaction in some people.

All in all, when it comes to food labels, let the buyer beware!

FAVORITE RECIPES

Please note that my previous book, *Dr. Rechtschaffen's Diet for Lifetime Weight Control and Better Health,* originally published in 1980, was published in a revised edition in April 1995. It contains more recipes than this book does, and it also provides a more complete eating plan if you are interested in a more formal diet.

Appetizers

BABA GHANNOUJ (EGGPLANT DIP)

A delicious spread that makes an excellent lunch, especially because it may be kept fresh in the refrigerator for several days. Serve with pita bread, raw vegetables, whole-grain French bread, or low-salt crackers.

- 1 large eggplant
- Juice of 1 lemon
- 1 tablespoon tahini or sesame paste
- 1 large clove garlic, minced
- 2 tablespoons chopped parsley
- 2 tablespoons olive oil

1. Cut stem and green hull from top of eggplant. Bake in oven for about 1 hour, or until very soft. Scoop pulp out of skin and mash thoroughly or press through a sieve.

2. Slowly beat lemon juice into eggplant alternately with sesame paste. Stir in garlic.

3. Pile into serving bowl and garnish with chopped parsley. Sprinkle with olive oil.

Yield: 4 servings.
Note: Some people like to sprinkle crushed red pepper on top.

BROILED MUSHROOMS

- 8 large fresh mushrooms
- 1 clove garlic, minced
- 2 teaspoons fresh chopped parsley or spinach leaves
- 2 teaspoons chopped chives or scallion tops
- 1 tablespoon chopped fresh dill or tarragon, or 1 teaspoon crumbled dry herb
- 1 tablespoon wine vinegar
- $1/4$ cup vegetable oil
- Freshly ground black pepper to taste

1. Remove stalks from mushrooms and reserve for soup stock. Wash mushrooms if necessary and dry on paper towel.

2. Combine remaining ingredients. Fill mushroom caps with mixture and arrange in small baking dish.

3. Broil 5 inches from source of heat until mushrooms are hot.

Yield: 4 servings.

TOMATO JUICE COCKTAIL

- 1 pint unsalted tomato juice
- 1 small onion, minced
- 2 tablespoons red wine vinegar
- 1 bay leaf
- $1/2$ teaspoon curry powder (optional)

1. Put all ingredients into a saucepan. Bring to a boil and simmer for 5 minutes.

2. Strain through a fine sieve lined with cheesecloth.

3. Chill and serve with a sprig of parsley. Pass the pepper grinder.

Yield: 2 servings.

Soups

The basis of most good soups is a savory stock made of chicken or fish with vegetables and herbs. Canned stocks and consommés are not recommended, not only because of their salt content but because their flavor is derived mainly from monosodium glutamate rather than from a complete protein food. (You may be able to find some acceptable prepared stock.) The two broths described here are indispensable, and the soups are perennial favorites.

SALT-FREE VEGETABLE BROTH

- 2 tablespoons vegetable oil
- 1 medium onion, chopped
- 1 clove garlic, chopped
- White part of 2 leeks, chopped, or 1 medium zucchini, diced
- 1 carrot, chopped
- $1/4$ cup parsley leaves
- 2 large fresh tomatoes, peeled or chopped, or
- 1-pound can salt-free whole tomatoes with liquid
- $1/2$ teaspoon coarsely cracked pepper
- 1 bay leaf
- 2 slices lemon
- $1/4$ teaspoon thyme
- 2 quarts water
- 1 cup dry white wine or dry vermouth

1. In heavy saucepan heat oil and sauté in it onion, garlic, leeks or zucchini, carrot, and parsley until onion is lightly browned.

2. Add tomatoes, pepper, bay leaf, lemon, thyme, water, and wine. Bring liquid to a boil, cover partially, and simmer for 40 minutes.

3. Strain broth. It will keep in refrigerator for 4 days. To keep for future use for soups and sauces, pour into freezer containers and freeze.

Yield: $1^1/2$ quarts.

SALT-FREE CHICKEN BROTH

This is the Chinese method of cooking a chicken. All the flavor is sealed in by means of the rapid boiling. The chicken meat is used for lunches. The bones are then returned to the soup kettle and long, slow cooking extracts all the flavor and gelatin from the bones. It's a way to have your chicken and eat it too!

- 4-pound roasting chicken, ready to cook
- 1 pound chicken wings, back, or necks
- 1 veal knuckle bone
- 2 carrots, halved
- 2 onions, one stuck with 3 cloves
- 2 leeks, white part only, sliced
- 1 clove garlic, halved
- Small bunch parsley stems
- $1/4$ teaspoon thyme
- 1 bay leaf
- 5 quarts water

1. A day in advance, combine all ingredients in a large soup kettle. Bring to a boil, skim off solids that rise to the surface, cover, and boil rapidly for 30 minutes.

2. Set soup off heat, uncover, and let cool to lukewarm. Remove chicken. Remove skin and meat from bones. Reserve chicken meat for lunches, and return skin and bones to soup kettle.

3. Return soup kettle to heat and bring to a boil. Simmer for 3 hours. Skim off every speck of fat from surface, strain through a sieve lined with cheesecloth, cool, then chill.

Yield: About 3 quarts.

Note: The broth will not keep long in the refrigerator due to the lack of salt. Freeze it in a container of suitable size or in ice cube trays. When cubes are frozen, remove them from trays and pack them in freezer bags. Return to freezer for use in soups and sauces.

GARDEN SOUP

- 10 ripe tomatoes, quartered
- 1 medium onion, sliced
- Handful of parsley sprigs
- 1 bay leaf
- 1 teaspoon peppercorns
- 4 cloves garlic
- Dash allspice
- ½ lemon, sliced
- ½ cup each shredded raw carrots and green pepper
- Unflavored yogurt
- ½ to 1 cup low-fat, low-salt chicken broth

1. Into large saucepan put chicken broth, tomatoes, onion, parsley, bay leaf, peppercorns, garlic, allspice, and lemon slices. Bring to a boil and simmer for 30 minutes. Add water to thin if necessary.

2. Press through fine sieve or strain to remove peppercorns and garlic cloves, and blend to smooth puree in electric blender.

3. Into puree stir shredded vegetables.

4. Serve hot with a topping of yogurt on each serving.

Yield: 4 servings.

GAZPACHO

- 2 firm, slim cucumbers
- 1 large sweet Bermuda onion
- 2 green peppers
- 8 red ripe tomatoes
- 2 large cloves garlic

- 6 tablespoons wine vinegar
- $1/4$ cup olive oil
- $1/2$ teaspoon coarsely cracked pepper
- $1^1/2$ cups ice water

1. Peel, seed, and finely dice 1 cucumber. Peel and finely chop half onion. Seed and sliver 1 green pepper. Peel, quarter, squeeze out seeds, and chop 6 tomatoes. Mince garlic.

2. Combine these prepared vegetables in bowl or pitcher and stir in vinegar, olive oil, pepper, and water. Chill for several hours.

3. Prepare garnish: Peel, seed, and dice remaining cucumber. Chop remaining onion. Seed and chop remaining green pepper. Peel, seed, and chop remaining tomatoes. Put each vegetable in separate bowl and refrigerate.

4. To serve, stir soup well and ladle into soup bowls. Pass chopped vegetables separately.

Yield: 6 servings.

Pasta

Marinara sauce is one of the basic components of any well-rounded diet. Rather than thinking of it only as a sauce for pasta, use it over baked potatoes, rice, fish, chicken, and many other foods instead of fatty sauces, butter, or sour cream. You can even use it as a braising liquid by thinning it with a little chicken broth, and bake fish or poultry in the sauce in a moderate oven.

SPAGHETTI WITH MARINARA SAUCE

- 2 tablespoons olive oil
- 1 large clove garlic, finely chopped
- 1 large (2 pound, 3 ounce) tin of Italian plum tomatoes
- ¼ can tomato paste
- ½ tablespoon basil
- ½ tablespoon oregano
- 1 pound spaghetti, preferably whole-grain
- 1 tablespoon chopped parsley
- Freshly ground black pepper

1. Heat oil in a heavy pot. Add peeled, chopped garlic and sauté for 3 to 4 minutes, being careful not to burn garlic.

2. Press tomatoes a few at a time through sieve into garlic and oil mixture. Stir frequently. When all tomatoes have been pressed through sieve, add remaining ingredients—except spaghetti, parsley, and pepper—and stir well.

3. Lower heat and simmer sauce for 45 minutes to 1 hour, stirring occasionally. Do not let sauce boil.

4. Cook spaghetti *al dente*, according to package instructions.

5. Pour sauce over freshly cooked hot spaghetti, sprinkle with parsley and pepper.

Yield: 6 servings.

LINGUINE WITH BROCCOLI

- 1 bunch broccoli, about 1¹/₄ pounds
- 4 tablespoons olive oil
- 2 teaspoons garlic, finely chopped
- ¹/₂ teaspoon crushed red pepper
- ¹/₂ cup chicken broth
- Freshly ground black pepper
- 1 pound linguine

1. Cut broccoli florettes off stems. Peel stems and cut into bite-size pieces. There should be about 6 cups of stem pieces and florettes.

2. Bring large pot of water to a boil and add broccoli. Cook about 1 to 3 minutes and drain. Do not overcook; broccoli must remain crisp. Run cold water over broccoli to chill quickly.

3. Heat oil in a skillet and add garlic. Cook briefly, without browning. Add broccoli and toss to heat through. Add crushed red pepper, broth, and ground black pepper to taste, and bring to a boil.

4. Cook linguine *al dente*, according to package directions.

5. Drain pasta and toss with hot broccoli mixture. Serve *immediately* on warm plates.

Yield: 6 servings.

Grains and Cereals

LEMON RICE

- 1¹/₂ cups water
- 1 cup rice
- 1 lemon
- 2 tablespoons vegetable oil
- ³/₄ cup low-fat buttermilk
- Chopped parsley

1. In saucepan combine water and rice and bring to a rapid boil. Cover with tight-fitting lid, reduce heat to lowest possible, and cook for 20 minutes.

2. While rice is cooking, remove thin yellow peel from lemon and sauté it in oil for 3 minutes. Discard rind, add buttermilk, and heat gently.

3. When rice is cooked and dry, remove cover and toss with fork. Stir in lemon-buttermilk mixture. Empty into serving dish and keep warm until ready to serve.

4. Sprinkle with parsley before serving.

Yield: 4 servings.

BULGUR PILAF

- 1 medium onion, chopped
- 2 cloves garlic, chopped
- 2 tablespoons vegetable or olive oil
- $^{1}/_{2}$ cup carrots, chopped
- $^{1}/_{2}$ cup celery, chopped
- 1 cup cracked wheat
- $^{1}/_{2}$ cup dry white wine
- 1 cup water

1. Sauté onion and garlic in oil until transparent, then add carrots and celery. Stir in cracked wheat, wine, and water. Bring to a boil, cover tightly, and cook over very low heat for about 1 hour, or until wheat is dry and cooked.

2. Fluff with a fork, cover partially, and keep over low heat for a few minutes before serving.

Yield: 4 servings.

Note: Bulgur pilaf can also be used to stuff a chicken or turkey.

Vegetables

RAW VEGETABLES
WITH COTTAGE CHEESE AND YOGURT

This recipe should be a standard "spur-of-the-moment" item in your list of choice dishes.

- ¹/₂ cucumber
- 2 radishes
- 4 scallions
- 1 pimento
- ¹/₂ cup low-salt, low-fat cottage cheese

- ¹/₂ cup low-salt, low-fat natural plain yogurt
- Freshly ground black pepper

1. Peel cucumber and discard seeds. Trim radishes and scallions.
2. Dice all the vegetables and place them in a decorative soup bowl.
3. Add cottage cheese and yogurt.
4. Sprinkle generously with freshly ground black pepper.
5. Stir gently so vegetables mix with cottage cheese and yogurt.

Yield: 1 serving. Serve with whole-grain crackers.
Variation: Fresh chopped tomato may be added.

POTATOES PAPRIKA

- 2 tablespoons vegetable oil
- 1 small onion, finely chopped
- 1 teaspoon sweet paprika
- 2 large potatoes, peeled and sliced $1/4$ inch thick

- 2 tablespoons vinegar
- 1 bay leaf
- $1/2$ teaspoon freshly ground black pepper

1. Heat oil in skillet, and sauté onion in it until golden.

2. Stir in paprika.

3. Add potatoes, vinegar, bay leaf, pepper, and enough water to barely cover the potatoes.

4. Cover skillet and cook over low heat for 30 minutes, or until potatoes are tender.

5. Serve pan sauce with potatoes.

Yield: 4 servings.

FRIED ONION RINGS

When you make these, make a lot. Pack what you can't eat in freezer bags and freeze.

- Large sweet or mild-flavored onions, peeled
- Buttermilk
- Unbleached flour
- Vegetable oil for deep frying

1. Slice onions about $1/8$ inch thick and separate into rings.
2. Soak rings in buttermilk for 1 hour. Drain well and dry between paper towels.
3. Shake a handful of onion rings at a time in a paper bag containing a little flour.
4. Remove onions and shake off excess flour. (A good way to do this is to place the floured rings in a collander, then shake collander over a piece of waxed paper; excess flour may be reused.)
5. In a thermostatically controlled fryer or electric wok, heat oil to 375 degrees. Fry a couple of handfuls of the floured rings at a time until golden and crisp.
6. Scoop rings out with slotted spoon onto a baking sheet lined with paper towels to drain.
7. Keep warm in a low oven until ready to serve.

To reheat, spread between thin aluminum foil sheets on a baking sheet and set into a 250-degree oven for 15 minutes.

Salads and Dressings

Everyone should eat salads frequently, and there is no better salad for everyday enjoyment than the traditional green salad tossed with homemade French Dressing, or Sauce Vinaigrette. Like marinara sauce, this vinaigrette dressing is an indispensable part of your overall eating plan. Its uses are unlimited.

FRENCH DRESSING, OR SAUCE VINAIGRETTE

- $1/4$ teaspoon freshly ground pepper
- $1/2$ teaspoon dry mustard
- 1 tablespoon vinegar or lemon juice
- 4 tablespoons salad oil (three parts safflower oil, 1 part olive oil)
- 1 clove garlic (optional)

1. In small bowl mix pepper and mustard with vinegar or lemon juice.
2. Gradually whip in salad oil, or blend all ingredients in a blender for a creamier texture.
3. The garlic may be used in either of two ways: Before putting salad greens in bowl, the bottom and sides may be rubbed with a garlic clove, cut in half. Or the garlic may be minced and added to the salad dressing.
4. Set dressing aside until ready to use. Whip again lightly before pouring over salad.

Yield: $1/3$ cup, or enough green salad to serve 4.

Note: If you want to reduce the fat content, dilute the dressing by adding 2 or 3 tablespoons of water. Blend together quickly and pour.

YOGURT DRESSING

- 8 ounces unflavored low-fat yogurt
- 1 tablespoon vegetable oil
- 1 tablespoon lemon juice or tarragon vinegar
- $1/2$ tablespoon mustard
- 1 tablespoon chopped chives
- 1 clove garlic, minced
- Freshly ground black pepper

Combine all ingredients and leave at room temperature until ready to spoon onto cold salad greens.

Yield: 4 servings.

BLENDER MAYONNAISE

- 1 egg
- $1/2$ teaspoon mustard
- 2 tablespoons vinegar
- 1 cup salad oil

1. Break egg into blender container. Add mustard and vinegar.
2. Add $1/4$ cup oil. Cover and turn to Low speed.
3. Immediately remove cover and pour in remaining $3/4$ cup oil in a steady stream.

Yield: $1^1/4$ cup ($1/5$ egg per quarter cup).

Homemade mayonnaise may be flavored to taste with garlic or herbs (try tarragon or dill, or basil and parsley for a different flavor) or curry (preferably paste rather than powder). Lemon juice may be used instead of vinegar. Red or white wine vinegar or cider vinegar may be used.

MIXED VEGETABLE SALAD

- 4 ripe tomatoes, peeled, seeded, and chopped
- 1 green pepper, seeded and chopped
- 1 cucumber, peeled, seeded, and diced
- 1 bunch radishes, sliced
- 1 bunch scallions, including tender green part, sliced
- $1/4$ cup chopped parsley
- 2 cups shredded romaine lettuce
- 1 clove garlic, minced
- Freshly ground black pepper, to taste
- 2 tablespoons lemon juice
- $1/3$ cup olive oil

1. Combine vegetables in salad bowl.
2. Add lemon juice and olive oil, and toss lightly.

Yield: 4 servings.

THREE-BEAN SALAD

- 1 19-ounce can white kidney beans
- 1 19-ounce can red kidney beans
- 1 19-ounce can chick peas (ceci)
- $1/2$ small red onion, diced
- 2 tablespoons fresh parsley, chopped

1. Pour beans and chick peas into collander and let juices wash away. Rinse thoroughly with cold water.
2. Place beans in large serving bowl.
3. Add onion and parsley.
4. Add Sauce Vinaigrette (see recipe on page 214).
5. Mix gently, chill, and serve.

Yield: 6 servings.

FRESH MEXICAN SALSA

- 1 medium tomato, chopped with skin
- ½ medium onion, chopped
- 6 sprigs fresh coriander, chopped (or ¼ teaspoon ground)

- 3 chilies, preferably serranos, chopped; do not seed
- ⅓ cup cold water

1. Mix chopped ingredients in a bowl.
2. Add water.

Yield: About 1½ cup.
Note: To retain flavors, best if made just before serving.

Meat, Poultry, and Fish

VEAL CHOPS IN WHITE WINE SAUCE

- 2 veal chops, about 8 ounces each, trimmed well
- 3 tablespoons vegetable oil
- 6 large fresh mushrooms, trimmed and sliced
- Coarsely cracked black pepper
- $^1/_2$ cup dry white wine
- 2 tablespoons dry sherry or Madeira
- 1 teaspoon cornstarch mixed with 1 tablespoon water

1. Sauté veal chops in the hot oil for about 3 minutes on each side, or until lightly browned.
2. Sprinkle mushrooms around chops and cook for 5 minutes, shaking pan frequently to toss the mushrooms in the oil.
3. Add pepper, white wine, and sherry or Madeira; cover, and braise over low heat for 5 to 10 minutes longer.
4. Remove chops to serving platter and keep warm.
5. Stir cornstarch mixture into liquid in pan and cook, stirring, for 1 minute, or until sauce is lightly thickened. Pour sauce and mushrooms over chops and garnish with parsley or watercress.

Yield: 2 servings.

GARLIC CHICKEN

- 2¹/₂- to 3-pound frying chicken, cut into serving portions
- Black pepper to taste
- 12 medium cloves garlic, peeled
- 1 onion, thinly sliced
- 3 carrots, thinly sliced
- 2 tablespoons chopped parsley
- ¹/₃ cup dry white wine
- 1 tablespoon dry sherry
- ¹/₃ cup unflavored low-fat yogurt

1. Preheat oven to 350 degrees.

2. Wash and dry chicken, and discard skin. Place chicken in a casserole dish and sprinkle with pepper, garlic cloves, onion, carrots, and parsley. Add wine and sherry. Cover tightly and bake in the preheated oven for 1¹/₂ hours, without raising the lid.

3. Remove casserole from oven and stir in yogurt.

4. The garlic cloves may be discarded, if desired; the flavor is in the chicken. Serve with rice or couscous.

Yield: 4 servings.

HERB-BROILED FISH STEAKS

- 2 8-ounce fish steaks (cod, swordfish, halibut, or salmon)
- 2 tablespoons vegetable oil
- 1 clove garlic, minced
- 2 tablespoons lemon juice
- $1/4$ teaspoon coarsely ground black pepper or to taste
- 1 teaspoon crumbled tarragon
- 2 tablespoons chopped green onions
- Lemon wedges

1. Preheat broiler and oil the broiler pan.

2. In small bowl mix oil, garlic, lemon juice, pepper, tarragon, and green onions. Spread half the mixture on the steaks, and arrange steaks on broiler pan.

3. Broil 5 to 6 inches from heat for 6 to 8 minutes. Turn steaks, spread with remaining tarragon mixture, and broil for 6 to 8 minutes longer, or until fish flakes easily.

Yield: 2 servings.

INDEX

acceptance, 28, 49, 72–73, 163–164
actinic keratosis, 101
activity. *See* mental activity; physical activity
adaptation, 3–4, 28
additives, food, 26, 32, 69, 97, 192, 194
adult-onset diabetes, 131
advertisements, food, 6, 117–118, 138, 189
aerobic activities, 23–24, 131
airplane meals, 97, 162
alcohol, 137
American Cancer Society, 50
American Heart Association, 55
anal itching, 105
anger, 91
antibiotics, natural, 34, 129
antioxidants, 181–182, 183
aphrodisiacs, 148–149
appetite
  decreasing, 16, 78
  insulin and, 76
  physical activity and, 59
appetizers, 199–200
  baba ghannouj (eggplant dip), 199
  mushrooms, broiled, 200
  in restaurants, 125–126

tomato juice cocktail, 200
apples, smoothie with bananas and, 134
applesauce, 92
arthritis, 74–75, 110, 157
artificial sweeteners, 26, 69
ascorbic acid, 100, 182
asthma, 34, 110
atherosclerosis, 63, 110
  food fiber and, 86
  salt intake and, 106–108
autoimmune disorders, 74–75

baba ghannouj (eggplant dip), 199
babies, 89, 135
balance, importance of, xviii, xx, xxi, 3–4, 13
bananas
  breakfast drink with strawberry and, 133
  smoothie with apples and, 134
beans, 33, 88
  three-bean salad, 216
beef, 87, 193
beef tallow, 159
beta-carotene, 33, 181–182, 187
beverages, 132–134

alcoholic, 137
apple-banana smoothie, 134
banana-strawberry breakfast drink, 133
coffee, 92, 97, 132
juices, 98, 200
orange-strawberry frappé, 134
soda, 83, 114, 115, 132
summertime breakfast drink, 133
tea, 92, 97
tomato juice cocktail, 200
see also water
binge eating, 5, 20–21, 91
birthday parties, 85
birth defects, 110
blender mayonnaise, 215
bloating, 104–105
blood clots, 34, 93, 157
blood flow, 17, 149
body fat
  inherited, 66–67
  physical activity and, 16–17, 19, 21, 23–24, 76, 89, 113
body type, 20
boredom, 19, 40, 80, 119
bran, 33–34, 35, 95, 102, 103, 105

ABOUT THE AUTHORS

Joseph S. Rechtschaffen, M.D., has been practicing medicine in New York City since 1950. He has served on the staffs of several hospitals, including New York Downtown, Beth Israel, and Flower Fifth Avenue, and currently has a private practice specializing in internal medicine and nutrition. He is the author, with Robert Carola, of *Dr. Rechtschaffen's Diet for Lifetime Weight Control and Better Health* (Kodansha, 1995). He lives in New York City.

Robert Carola is a freelance writer who has cowritten several college textbooks, including *Human Anatomy and Physiology*, Third Edition (McGraw Hill, 1995). He is the coauthor of the updated edition of *Dr. Rechtschaffen's Diet for Lifetime Weight Control and Better Health* (Kodansha, 1995), and has also written for many corporate clients, including IBM, Exxon, and Michigan Bell.